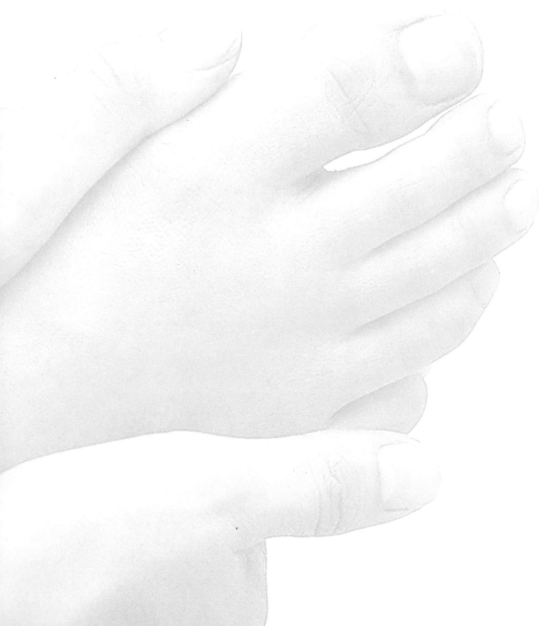

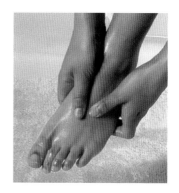

home spa
feet

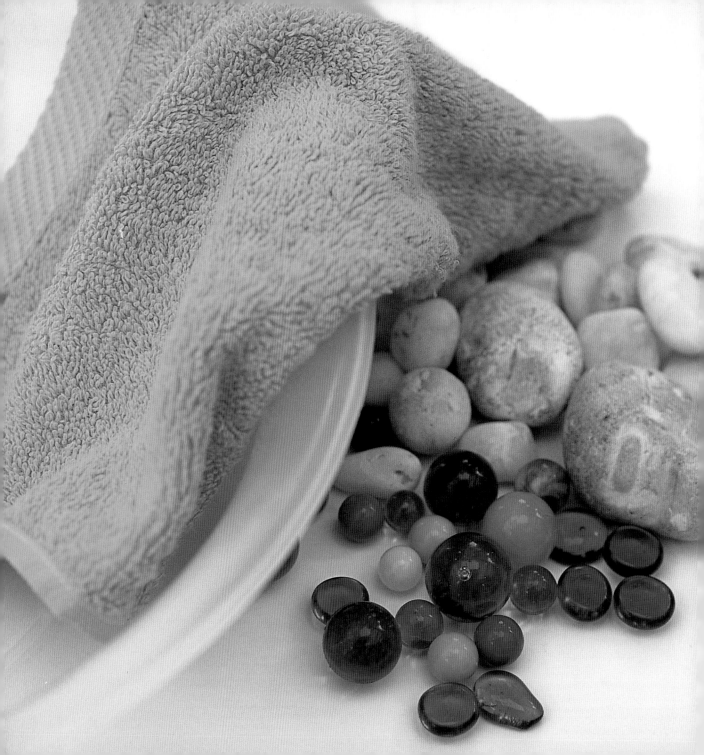

home spa
feet

Soothe and revive tired feet with
simple indulgences, including
soaking, scrubs, moisturizing,
reflexology and foot massage

Tracey Kelly

LORENZ BOOKS

This edition is published by
Lorenz Books

Lorenz Books is an imprint of
Anness Publishing Ltd
Hermes House,
88–89 Blackfriars Road,
London SE1 8HA
tel. 020 7401 2077;
fax 020 7633 9499
www.lorenzbooks.com;
info@anness.com

© Anness Publishing Ltd 2004

UK agent:
The Manning Partnership Ltd,
6 The Old Dairy, Melcombe
Road, Bath BA2 3LR;
tel. 01225 478444; fax 01225
478440; sales@manning-
partnership.co.uk

UK distributor:
Grantham Book Services Ltd,
Isaac Newton Way, Alma Park
Industrial Estate,
Grantham, Lincs NG31 9SD;
tel. 01476 541080; fax 01476
541061; orders@gbs.tbs-ltd.co.uk

North American agent/distributor:
National Book Network, 4501
Forbes Boulevard, Suite 200,
Lanham, MD 20706;
tel. 301 459 3366; fax 301 429
5746; www.nbnbooks.com

Australian agent/distributor:
Pan Macmillan Australia,
Level 18, St Martins Tower,
31 Market St, Sydney, NSW
2000; tel. 1300 135 113;
fax 1300 135 103;
customer.service@macmillan.
com.au

New Zealand agent/distributor:
David Bateman Ltd, 30 Tarndale
Grove, Off Bush Road, Albany,
Auckland; tel. (09) 415 7664;
fax (09) 415 8892

A CIP catalogue record for
this book is available from the
British Library.

Publisher: Joanna Lorenz
Editorial Director: Helen Sudell
Project Editor: Catherine Stuart
Designer: Louise Clements
Production Controller: Claire Rae
Editorial Reader: Hayley Kerr

10 9 8 7 6 5 4 3 2 1

NOTE
The author and publishers have made every effort to ensure that all
instructions within this book are accurate and safe, and cannot accept
liability for any resulting injury, damage or loss to persons or property,
however it may arise. If you do have any special needs or problems,
consult your doctor or a physiotherapist. This book cannot replace
medical consultation and should be used in conjunction with
professional advice.

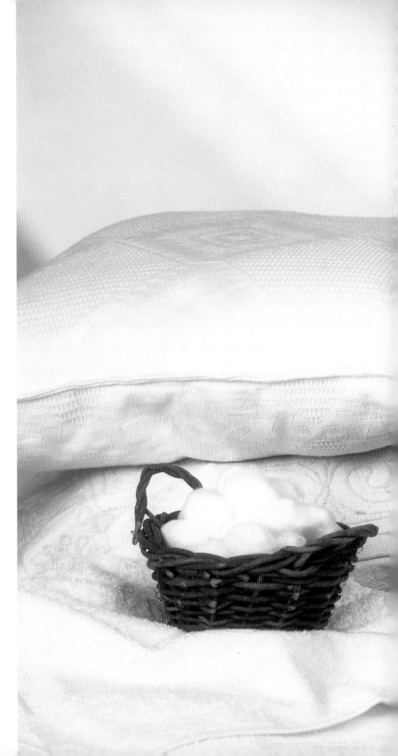

contents

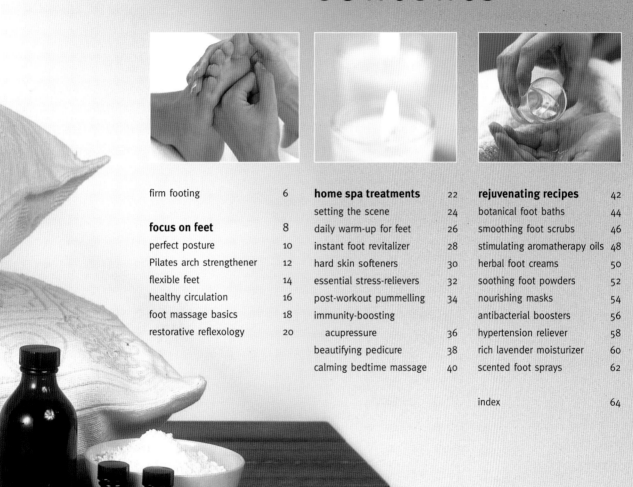

firm footing

During your lifetime, your feet may carry you the equivalent of five times around the globe. So it makes sense to put a little time aside to care for them on a daily basis.

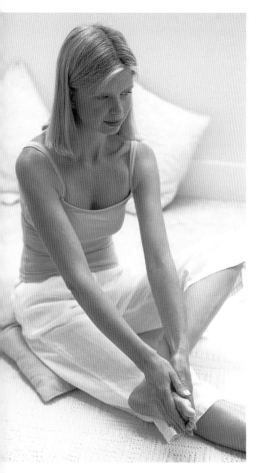

In this book, we will look at ways in which you can improve the health and condition of your feet. One of the best places to start is with comfortable footwear, to give good stability and let your feet breathe. Your feet support and balance your whole body, so regular foot care and good posture play a vital role in reducing wear and tear.

everyday care

It is important to warm up the muscles with simple stretches before strenuous activity, treatment or prolonged standing. A few simple exercises each morning can increase the strength and flexibility of the feet, helping to prevent injury and strain.

Pilates recognizes the importance of feet in distributing body weight, devising gentle moves which seek to create a line of strength from the toes upwards and re-align the neck, spine and hips.

rejuvenating therapies

A massage session – either self-applied or with the help of a partner – is a great way to rejuvenate the feet while relaxing the rest of the body. This, and other well-practised arts such as reflexology and acupressure, have long made use of the feet as instruments of holistic healing. A range of gentle exercises are included in the following pages to help combat muscular strain and fatigue while boosting resilience and vitality.

above Caring for your feet improves suppleness and helps to prevent pain.

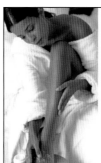

treat your feet

- Moisturize the feet regularly – especially the heels, ankles, pads on the sides and base of the toes.
- Walk in the sand when you can – this is great for conditioning muscles in the legs and feet.
- Paddle in the sea when you can, or run cold water over the feet to stimulate circulation.
- Use sunscreen: the feet also need protecting against UV rays.

new vitality

Rediscover sensation in your feet by trying a range of regular foot treatments. Mini-massages and circulation boosters help to keep feet supple, while soaking and scrubbing softens the soles and floods them with new life. Cooling down after sport is important, too. Follow tips on squeezing and relieving muscles to counter all the stresses of a workout.

Feet on top form deserve a treat; a pedicure is the perfect way to beautify healthy toes. It's easy to shape toenails and master smudge-free polishing using just a few simple techniques.

pure pampering

Commercial massage oils, lotions and scrubs can be expensive and may contain harmful chemicals. You can make pure cosmetics at home using a few accessible ingredients. Adding fragrant flower and herb essences to creams, masks and powders conditions the skin and tissues, while giving a lift to the spirits. Aromatic massage and moisturizing blends are easily made by mixing carrier oils with essential oils.

right *Foot massage not only feels good, it helps keep the feet in top condition.*

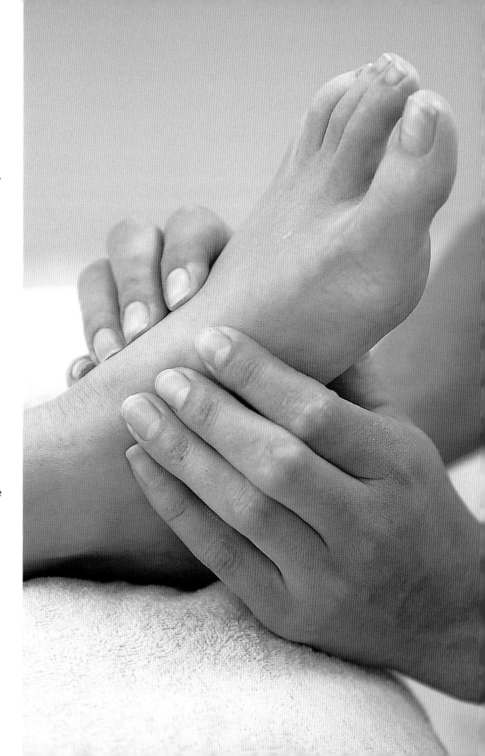

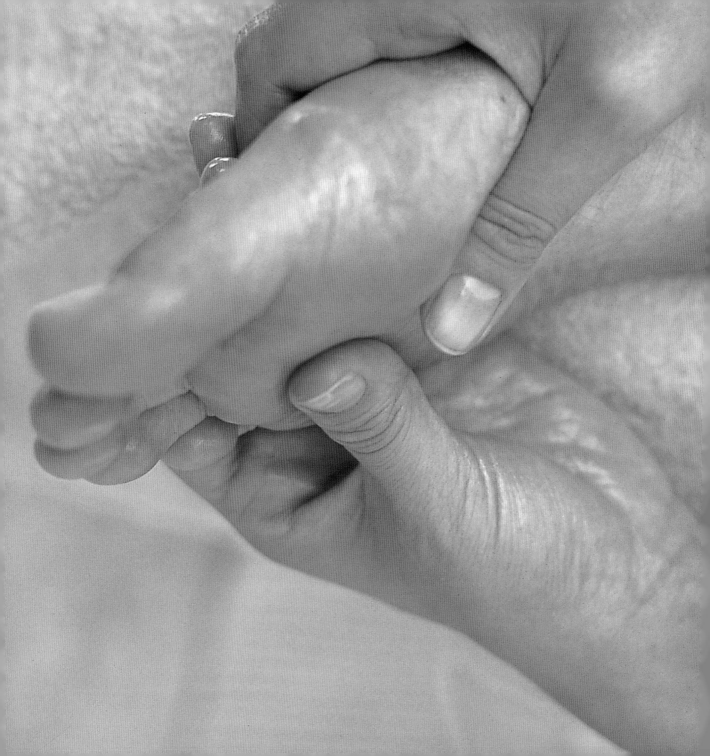

focus on feet

Rejuvenate your body from the toes upwards by putting feet first. You can enjoy feeling energized and refreshed every day by ensuring the feet remain supple and smooth, and by trying out basic routines incorporating foot massage, stretching, Pilates and reflexology.

perfect posture

The whole body is affected by the way we stand, walk and sit. Poor posture places
undue stress on the body's joints, and projects a negative self-image to the world.

Holding yourself incorrectly can create health problems such as lower back pain, headaches and shoulder aches. It can also affect nerve function and spinal alignment, making you appear older. So if your posture needs help, it is a good idea to practise improving it now, so that standing tall becomes as natural as breathing.

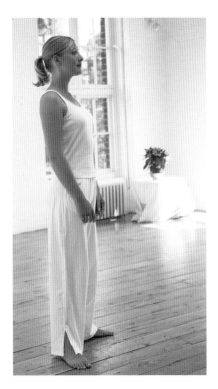

above *Correct posture relieves stress on the joints and improves your appearance.*

sensible shoes

The type of shoes you wear significantly affects your posture. Constant wearing of high-heeled or stiletto shoes squashes the balls of the feet into an unnatural position until, over time, the toes are likely to become deformed. The upper body is pushed forwards, throwing spinal alignment into disarray and forcing the hips, knees and calves to carry a disproportionate amount of body weight.

For this reason, podiatrists recommend wearing shoes that allow the feet room to expand when you walk. Shoes for daily wear should not have heels that are more than 4cm / 1$\frac{1}{2}$in high. Look for a wide base and a soft, spongy sole to absorb the shock of your weight on pavements. You should also check your size when buying a new pair of shoes. Many adults take at least a shoe size bigger than they did as teenagers.

standing proud

The following exercise is an excellent way to check your posture. Wearing shoes that support the arches in your feet, begin by standing with your head up straight and your chin tucked in. Keep your shoulder blades level, your hips equal and symmetrical, the knees facing forwards and the abdominals strong. Now lift your chin a little and begin lengthening through the spine, imagining that your body can rise up until your head touches the ceiling. Keep your pelvis steady; don't let it tilt backwards or forwards. This is the correct standing position and should be practised whenever you are stationary.

If you need help in attaining good posture for activities such as sitting at a desk, walking, carrying objects and playing instruments, practitioners of the Alexander technique and Feldenkrais method can help. Disciplines such as yoga and t'ai chi are also wonderful ways to improve balance. To learn more about the role of the feet in correcting posture, try the following exercises.

spreading toes and defining arches

Compare these profiles to see how the toes can be positioned to spread body weight evenly through the whole foot, improving the alignment of the ankles, hips and knees.

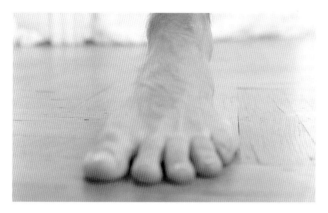

above: **Correct** – *the ankle is in the middle of the foot, with the toes distributing weight evenly across the ball and heel.*

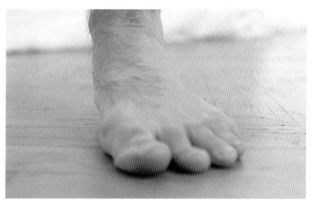

above: **Incorrect** – *the ankle bone is leaning inwards, collapsing the arch and placing strain on the inside of the knee.*

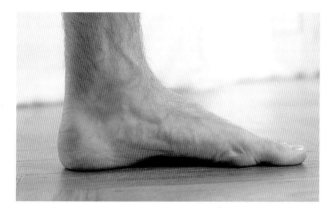

above: **Correct** – *the foot muscles are maintaining the arch and holding the ankle in the centre of the foot.*

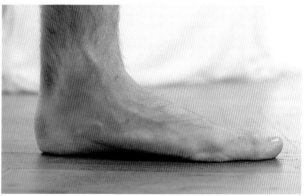

above: **Incorrect** – *the natural arch of the foot has all but disappeared, causing the ankle to roll inwards.*

pilates arch strengthener

If your arches are weak, then walking – not to mention exercise – will be awkward. This Pilates set can help to strengthen your arches, improving stability and balance.

Perform the following exercise in your bare feet, preferably on a vinyl or wooden floor, or use a stable exercise mat. Lift and lower several times to get the posture right.

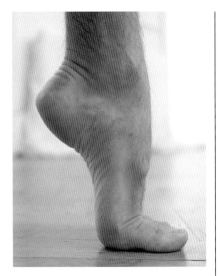

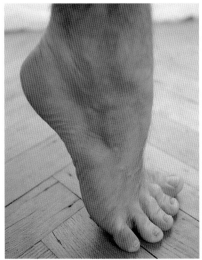

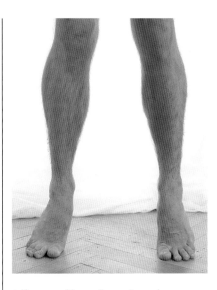

1 Stand with the feet facing forwards, aligned with your hips. Gradually rise up on to tiptoes and perch there for a few seconds, aiming to lift the heels directly above the balls of the big toes. Make sure that the ankles do not fall to the left or right. This move helps to stimulate the feet, stretch the arches and strengthen the line from the foot through the ankle, to the knee and hip.

2 The next time you perch on tiptoes, spread your toes wide to form a firm base, pressing them down to help you balance. When you have risen up and down on your toes enough to be familiar with the action, concentrate on going straight up on to tiptoes, trying not to lean forwards each time you lift. You will feel an immediate stimulation in the arches of the feet.

3 If your ankles collapse inwards, as shown here, try extending your little toes outwards to restore balance and tilt the ankles back in line with the centre of the body. If your ankles fall outwards, extend the big toes forward as far as possible, pressing them into the floor, to anchor the ball of the foot and provide a stable support for the legs and ankles.

right *Feet provide support and stability for the entire body during exercise and dance, so it is important for arches to be strong and flexible. Pilates helps to reshape the arches via a combination of stretching and balancing.*

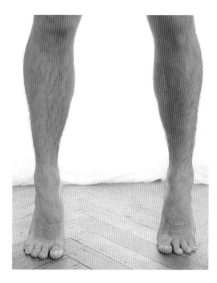

4 When both ankles are over the ball of the foot, push your ankle forwards a little more, if you can, to increase the stretch in your arches. With each of these steps, it doesn't matter if you can't get your heels as high as those pictured here. As long as you can maintain your balance on tiptoes, and feel the stretch throughout your foot, you will begin to strengthen and reshape your arches.

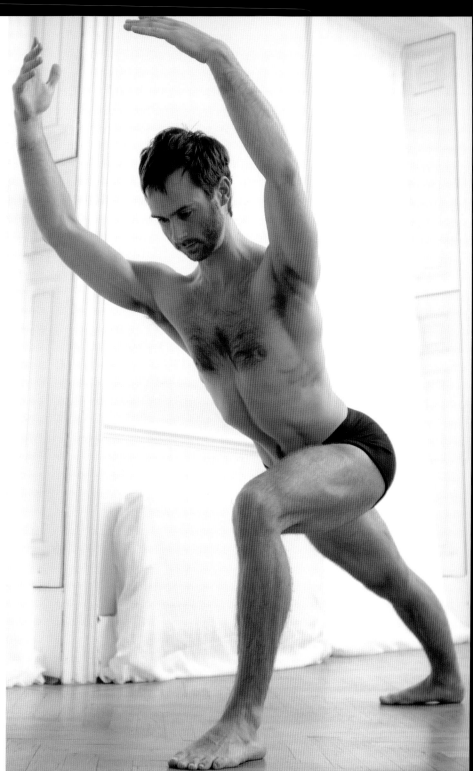

flexible feet

By doing quick, simple stretches in the morning, during the day and before bed, you can minimize the chance of injuries and cramp in the lower legs, ankles and feet.

energizing stretch

This is a very useful way to invigorate the quadricep muscles at the front of the leg and send blood coursing through the calf and foot.

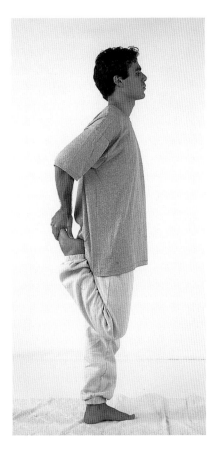

First, stand on one leg, bending the other leg behind you. Clasp the foot with your hand and pull it further into your buttocks. Relax and repeat with the other leg. This simple leg stretch can be practised almost anywhere. Try it during your coffee break at work and see how quickly energy returns to the legs and upper body.

Calf and foot stretches such as this are also immensely beneficial on long-haul flights where you are forced to sit in the same position for hours at a time. Go to the back of the cabin, stand for a few moments to get your bearings, and then do the stretch, taking care to steady yourself against a surface with one hand in case of sudden turbulence.

left Calf and foot stretches energize the lower legs by allowing blood to flow more freely. They are a particularly useful antidote to sedentary, office-based work.

quick calf and foot stretch

These stretches can be performed lying on a bed if it is more comfortable.

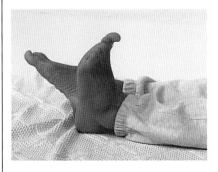

1 Sit on the floor with both legs straight out in front of you, then alternately flex and extend each foot.

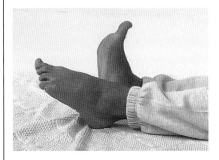

2 Make sure that one foot is flexed while the other is extended and vice versa.

dancing steps

A highly aerobic activity, dancing wakes up the system in no uncertain terms – and it elevates your mood and helps prevent stress while improving the look and tone of your legs and feet.

Dance has developed in all world cultures as a celebration of life and self-expression, and there are many forms to choose from. Many gyms offer classes in various styles, such as salsa, samba, ceroc, jazz and ballroom. You may want to choose a highly vigorous form, such as Latin American dance; or one that is lower key, such as free-form, ballroom or line dancing.

Some complex dance routines – such as those found in Indian and Indonesian classical forms, and Western ballet – will keep your mind occupied with their very intricate moves, while keeping you on your toes – literally. The benefits extend beyond the lower body, too. As well as ensuring legs and feet remain in top condition, Egyptian belly dancing (*raqs sharqi*) is great for toning muscles in the midriff, shoulders and arms.

right *Dance techniques – whether intricately choreographed or free-form – condition the feet and are great fun.*

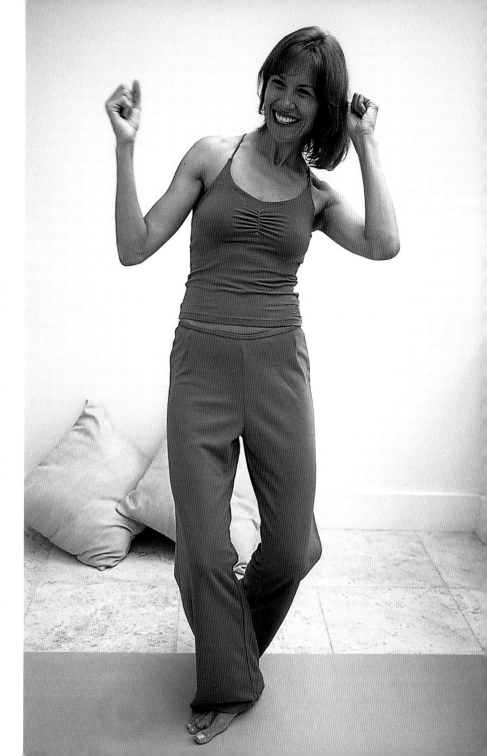

healthy circulation

Exercise and basic foot care will help to keep your feet warm and healthy. Use these guidelines to promote good circulation throughout the day, whatever the weather.

If you suffer from cold feet, there are many possible causes. It may be that your shoes are too tight, or that you're wearing socks too thick to allow the feet to breathe, cutting off the circulation. Choose shoes spacious enough to allow air-flow around the toes, and socks made from cotton, wool and silk or natural fabric/nylon blends.

warming cold feet

On winter days, it is worth warming up the feet before putting boots on, or they are likely to stay cold all day. Try running very warm water over your feet and then patting them dry with a towel, making sure to remove any excess moisture.

Moisturizing the feet as a matter of course is another great way of promoting blood flow while improving their general condition. You can also try a few simple foot flexes, like those described earlier, or a mini-massage, so that feet are warm and lively by the time you begin walking.

circulation jump-start

Stand on a couple of cushions and try to balance. Move your feet, one at a time, in a walking motion for about five minutes. Now use alternate feet to step up on to the cushions. Do 10 steps with one foot and then repeat with the other.

These moves work all the muscles in the leg and hip joints, and enhance the flow of blood through the feet. They also reduce swelling. By sitting down all day and keeping feet in the same position, blood swells feet and causes circulation to become sluggish.

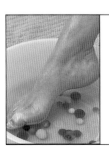

circulation-booster foot bath

- Half-fill a foot bowl with warm water, and then add a layer of marbles of different sizes. Pour in 5ml / 1 tsp of essential oil – mandarin is particularly useful for circulatory problems.
- Push the feet backwards and forwards over the marbles, so that the length of the sole is stimulated. Remove feet and dry.

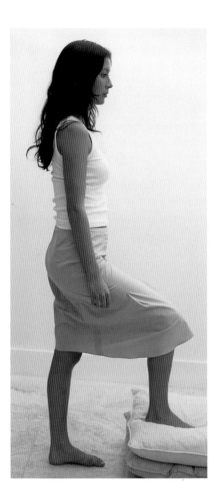

above *Stepping on cushions is a gentle, effective way to boost circulation.*

inverted legs pose

This modified yoga pose is an excellent tonic for restless legs and feet, which may occur in the evening if the body has been sedentary for most of the day.

Place a folded blanket or rug on the floor, along with a cushion to support your head and neck. Get into position by first sitting down with one buttock side-on to the wall. Then ease your upper body down towards the floor, at the same time raising your legs so that they are supported in an upright fashion against the surface of the wall.

The back of your legs should be flat against the wall, with the seat of your buttocks nestled snugly into the angle it forms with the floor. The upper body should be straight and relaxed. Release the tension from your arms, close your eyes and allow your mind to wander away from the events of the day.

Remain in this position for up to 15 minutes, after which time you should come back to an upright position by sliding the legs slowly down the wall, folding them at one side of your body as you gently swivel back around to centre.

right *This yoga-inspired pose can help to ease restless leg syndrome.*

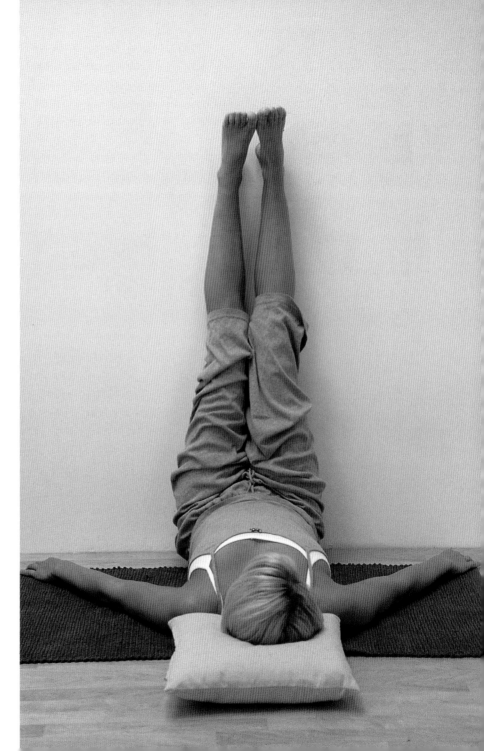

foot massage basics

By using just a few simple strokes, you can perform a great foot massage on yourself and others. Try these easy-to-learn techniques to get familiar with the basics.

When first learning foot massage, it is a good idea to practise on your own feet, in order to gauge the various levels of comfort and pressure. You can then use the same strokes on a partner or friend. Essential oils are a useful addition to any treatment – the scents will work in harmony with the strokes to stimulate nerves and nourish skin.

getting ready

First, wash your hands and check that your nails are trimmed. It is a good idea to cleanse the feet before massage. Try adding two drops of lavender oil and one drop of tea tree oil to some warm water in a basin or tub. This excellent aromatic cleanser relaxes the whole body with its scent while working to keep the feet soft and supple.

You will need to find a comfortable position, in a warm and quiet area, free from interruptions. The feet – your own or those of the recipient – should be where you can reach them without twisting or bending. If treating yourself, you might opt to rest the foot on your knee, or to sit on the floor with the leg bent towards you. If treating a friend,

right Elevating the feet for massage improves access and effectiveness.

they might prefer to sit upright in a chair or to lie on the floor, resting their head and neck on a flat pillow.

The legs should be supported by a stool of suitable height, with the knees slightly bent to aid circulation. If you wish, you can place a towel beneath the calves for added comfort and to prevent spillages if working with oils.

pressure and health

Note that the sensitivity of the feet can vary at different times and with different people. To test responses to speed and pressure, start with a very light touch and gradually increase to tolerance. As a rule, fast strokes are energizing, while slower, rhythmic strokes promote calm. Firm pressure helps to release muscular tension, and a gentler touch to soothe.

Do not massage feet infected by athlete's foot or verrucas. Treat with 3 drops of thyme oil blended with 5ml / 1 tsp carrier oil.

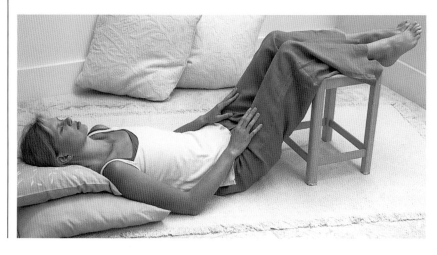

The following exercises introduce you to some of the core strokes used in foot massage. These are very basic movements designed to help you achieve a firm, but gentle pressure, and are suitable for use on your own feet or those of a partner.

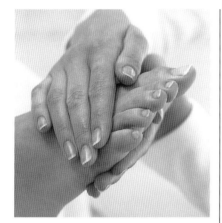

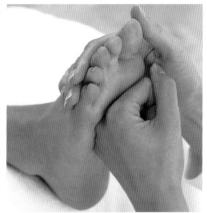

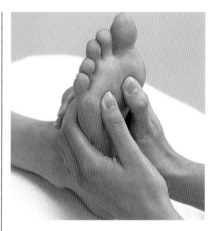

effleurage, or stroking

Use this stroking movement to start and finish all mini-massages – "book-ending" a foot massage in this way completes the energy circuit and rounds off the treatment. To perform the move, gently sandwich the foot between your palms, so that the fingers are resting across the base of the toes. Slide the fingers down the foot on both sides, from the toe joints to the heel and shin, and then back up to the starting point. Repeat this movement two or three times, gradually increasing pressure each time, until you feel a stimulation in the feet.

knuckling

This simple move is good for warming the muscles and for releasing tension after a strenuous workout or when stress has tightened the muscles in general. Make a loose "fist" with the flat part of your fingers, keeping the knuckles and joints at right angles with the palm, and press it into the ball of the foot. Work the knuckles up and down the base of this foot, rotating the "fist" a little as you go. Be sure to cover the entire sole of the foot, from heel to toe, so that the whole area is loosened and warmed by the movements.

thumb circling

To treat the small, fleshy areas of the foot, begin by placing the thumbs on the ball of the foot, one slightly higher than the other. Now use the pads of your thumbs to massage the whole of this area, making small, rotational movements. Alternate the two thumbs until you get a rhythm going; this is a bit like playing an instrument by ear – you will be able to "feel" how much pressure to apply and how fast to go. This technique warms the tissues and nerve-endings, stimulating circulation and reviving tired and tense feet.

restorative reflexology

After warming up with a foot massage, why not try a little healing reflexology? This holistic practice uses stimuli on the feet to direct healing energies through the body.

Reflexologists believe that the feet hold a "map" of the body, with every organ represented by a point, or "reflex", on either the toes, soles, heels, tops or sides. Although it sounds a complex procedure, basic reflexology moves are easy to perform at home, and are just as restorative for general health as for specific ailments.

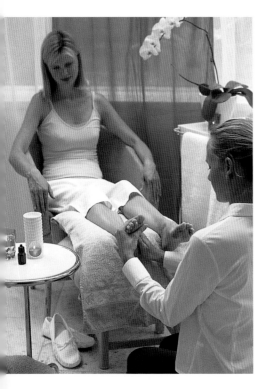

above *To create an air of serenity, keep harsh light and outside noise at bay.*

balancing and healing

Reflexology is based on two important principles: that the body has an innate ability to heal itself, and that small parts of the body can be used to treat the whole system. As a result of illness, stress or injury, the systems of the body are thrown out of balance and its vital energy pathways are blocked. The body begins to cry for help, which shows up in various ways – headaches and mood swings, for example – and toxins build up around the relevant reflex points.

Reflex points on the feet where toxic deposits develop may feel sensitive and painful. They may also feel hard, tight or suffused with little grains. By stimulating these points with massage, the previous congestion is eased and this frees up energy blockages in corresponding places elsewhere in the system, encouraging the body to rebalance and heal itself.

treatment with reflexology

Find a comfortable position for the person whose feet you are treating. They may wish to sit on the floor, leaning against firm, bulky cushions, or to sit in an armchair with an upright chair or stool of a suitable height to support their legs. Whichever position is chosen, make sure that their back, neck and head are fully supported so as not to place the spine under strain, and that their knees are bent so that the circulation can flow freely. Have a blanket on hand for warmth, as well as some fresh towels – one to place under the feet and one or two to keep the feet warm.

Start by massaging your partner's feet to warm and relax the tissues, including a gentle rotation of the ankles. This stimulates the receiver's blood supply so that the reflex points can respond fully. Use massage to link one reflex movement to the next.

After you've covered the reflex points, it is a good idea to end your treatment by giving another gentle massage, to instil a sense of relaxation.

The following exercises will show you how different actions may be used to stimulate reflexes on the foot. Generally, the level of pressure applied to the bony areas of the feet should be lighter than that applied to fleshier parts like the heel or ball.

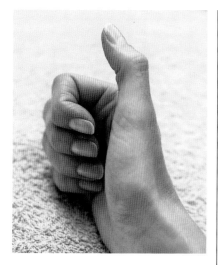

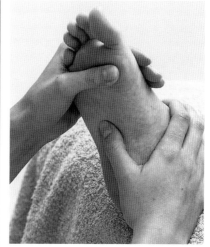

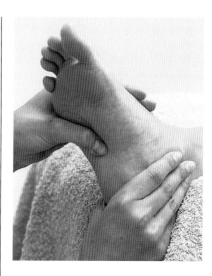

thumb walking or crawling

Holding your thumb straight up in front of you, bend it from the first joint and straighten it again. By repeating this movement as you rest on the skin, thumb-walk across the area, moving up and down, feeling the surface beneath the thumb. This movement resembles a caterpillar crawling across the ground. It is often used in reflexology to aid the uptake of nutrients by the digestive system and small intestine.

rotation on a point

This action is used for sensitive reflexes such as the zone related to the adrenal glands, located on the inner arch of the left foot. Place the pad of your thumb on the reflex point, and with your holding hand, flex the foot slowly into the thumb. Rotate the foot in a circular movement around the thumb. Try exerting more pressure, a little bit at a time. Make sure you get feedback on the comfort levels from the recipient, and ease off directly if you feel you've pressed too hard.

pinpoint, or hooking

This action is used for smaller reflexes, such as the gall bladder at the centre of the sole, or for those difficult to locate, such as the ureter, which runs from the arch to the heel. With your hand in mid-air, move the thumb and fingers together and apart like a pincer. Place your hand on the foot and, with the inner part of the thumb, apply pressure to the point and hold. Keep the pressure steady as you hook in the thumb, then move this digit back to its original position.

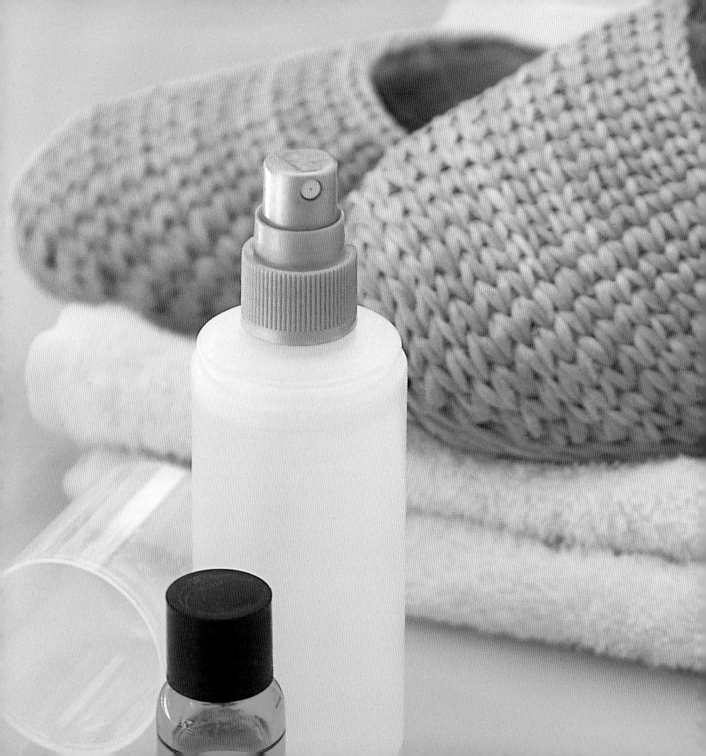

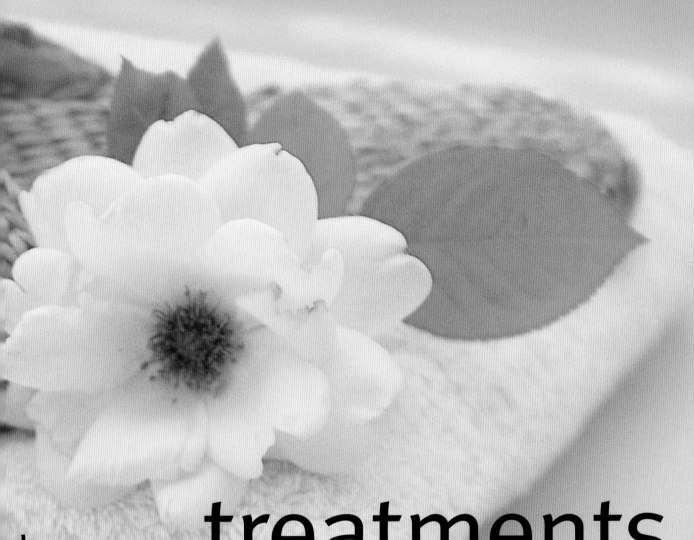

home spa treatments

Transform your feet with this comprehensive range of foot therapies, from a 5-minute warm-up massage to stress-busting exercises, hard skin softeners and essential pedicure tips. Create a sumptuous spa in your bathroom or practise revitalizing treatments during a break from work.

setting the scene

Create an oasis for treatment by setting aside a quiet room or corner where you can fully concentrate on making yourself – or a friend – feel really pampered.

Beautiful surroundings make for restful, happy feelings, which aid any grooming or health-giving treatment you undertake. First, tidy up clutter and turn off the ringer on the telephone, so that you are not distracted by outside concerns. Make sure the room is warm but not hot, as cooler temperatures are healthier for the whole system.

gather simple tools

Turn off harsh, overhead lights, opting for a soft, candlelit environment instead. Add a vase full of fresh, fragrant flowers to lift the spirits, and if you desire, play some very simple instrumental music with a slow to medium beat.

Gather together the tools required for the treatment you are planning to carry out. For massage, have two clean towels ready: one to put under the feet and another to cover them. Place massage oils on a tray or small table in case they spill. Keep a pot of moisturizing lotion nearby for post-treatment pampering, and have a pair of comfortable slippers ready to warm treated feet.

If you are carrying out reflexology, you may need a little powder to rub between your hands in case they get sticky or clammy. If you plan to work on the floor, lay down a foam exercise mat. When propping up the feet of a partner, you can use either a small stool or large scatter pillows. Experiment to see which is the more comfortable for you.

patch testing with oils

Before using an essential oil, test for skin sensitivity. Mix two drops with 1 tsp carrier oil, then massage into the skin on your elbow. If there's no reaction within six hours, it is safe to use. If the skin becomes irritated, apply more carrier oil to neutralize the effect.

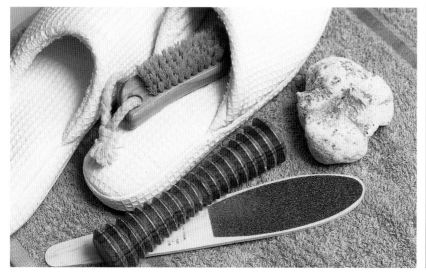

left *A pumice stone, brush and foot massager are ideal for treating the feet.*

right *A home spa provides a sanctuary where you can relax with friends.*

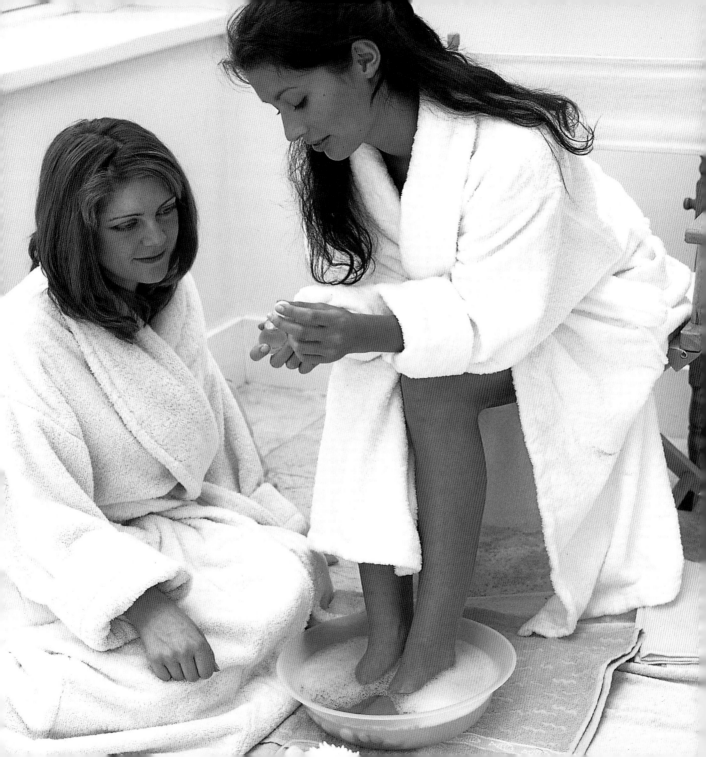

daily warm-up for feet

Start your day fresh and alert with these invigorating warm-up massages, which relax
the muscles and stimulate circulation, reawakening energy in your feet.

This fast, effective self-massage is ideally carried out just after you hop out of the
shower. Choose a favourite cream or diluted essential oil to apply to the feet.

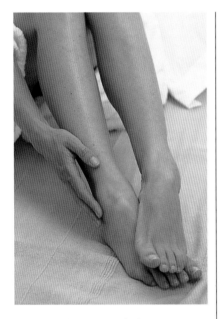 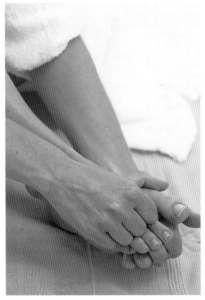 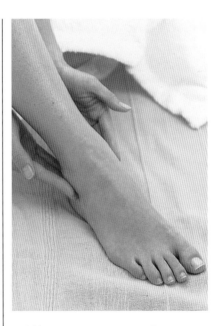

1 Use your fingers to rub the cream or
oil liberally over the top of the right
foot. Then position your left foot on
top, and use the sole to massage this
whole area a little more. Apply heavier
pressure to the toes of the right foot,
than to the ankle area, as they are
less delicate.

2 Now use your hands to smooth the
cream or massage oil all over the toes.
Make fists with both hands, placing
the left hand underneath so that the
knuckles support the toes, and the
right fist on top. Slide the knuckles
across each toe in turn, working left to
right, using firm pressure.

3 Add more cream to your palms,
ensuring an even spread. Massage
both areas of the ankle, making three
distinct rotations, starting in a
clockwise direction. Repeat with
anticlockwise rotations. If your ankles
still feel tense, perform a second set
of rotations in both directions.

right *For a useful morning stretch, sit with the feet in front of you, then wiggle all of your toes to wake up circulation. Next, stretch the toes towards the ceiling for a few seconds, so that the balls of the feet protrude, then allow to relax again.*

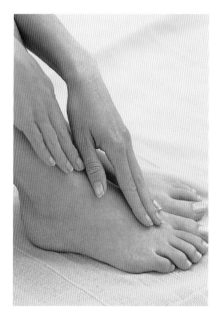

4 Replenish the cream or oil on your palms again, then use alternate hands to stroke the top of the foot, starting from the toes and working towards the ankle. Begin with a very light touch to warm up, then gradually increase the pressure in each new movement to kick-start circulation.

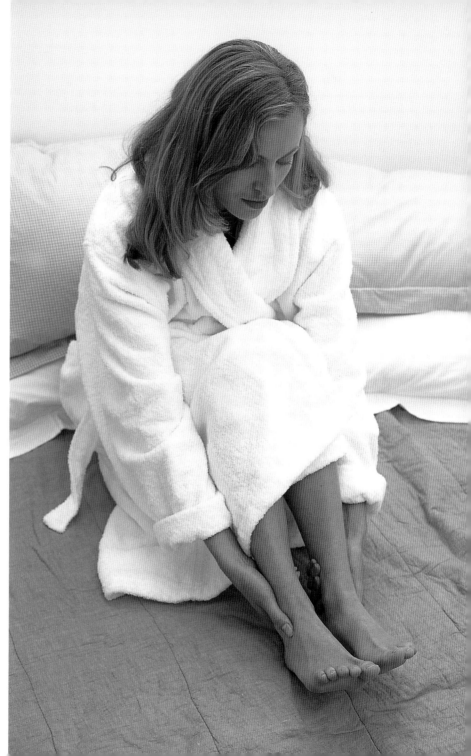

instant foot revitalizer

A mini-massage can provide instant benefits for tired feet. This massage is best done with a partner, and you can swap places so that you both reap the rewards.

If desired, blend a small amount of massage oil with a few drops of peppermint or juniper essential oil, and rub between the palms. These oils stimulate and warm.

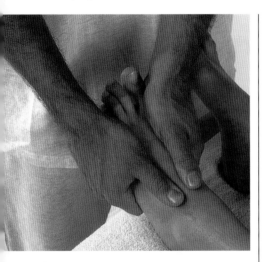
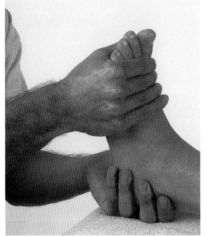
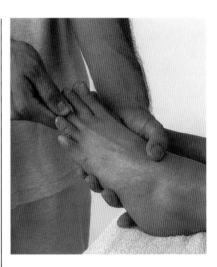

1 Hold the foot in your hands, with thumbs on top and fingers underneath. Gently stretch across the top of the foot, aiming to keep your fingers still while moving your thumbs. This technique is known as spreading. It is useful for warming tight tendons and muscles that may have been over-stretched during a workout, a running session or simply a day's worth of weight and strain on the feet.

2 Flex the foot, pushing against the resistance to loosen the whole foot and ankle a little. Now gently extend the foot, stretching it as far as is comfortable. Next, twist the foot gently, using a wringing motion, in both directions to stretch the muscles in every way. This technique loosens the muscles and prevents cramps from developing in the joints.

3 Hold one of the toes between thumb and forefinger and give the tip a gentle squeeze, followed by a pulling action. Repeat this action for all toes. Begin this action gently – you don't want to break the toes! – and feel your way to the correct level of pulling and stretching you can safely carry out. Toes are often cramped in shoes all day without moving, and this action helps keep them flexible.

right *After a hard day, you can sit back and enjoy the benefits of a five-minute foot massage, perfect for soothing tired and overworked feet, and for relieving muscular aches and tensions in the lower legs.*

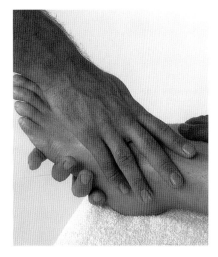

4 Support the foot with one hand and place the other one over the top, extending the fingers to cover the whole of this upper side. Stroke the upper side with the other hand. Smoothly stroke all the way from the toes to the ankle. Repeat all the movements on the other foot. This soothing action stimulates the circulation and draws the energy back upwards, towards the heart.

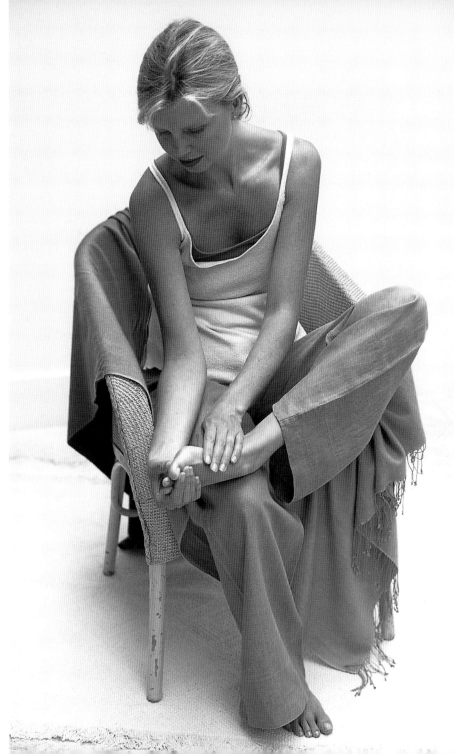

hard skin softeners

The secret of dealing with hard skin is to rub it gently every day, rather than trying to remove it all in one session – otherwise you may risk having irritated, red feet.

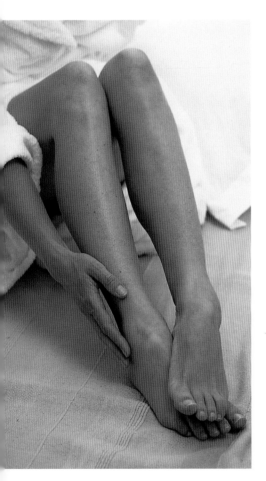

above To keep feet beautiful, pamper them as you would your hands.

The following foot-care routine, if performed daily or every other day, should keep your feet supple and smooth and guard against build-up of hard skin and calluses.

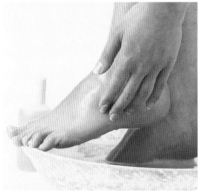

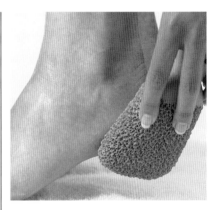

1 Start your softening routine by soaking the feet in a bowl of warm, slightly soapy water to cleanse and make them more pliable. If the skin on the soles has become very rough, add 30ml / 2 tbsp bicarbonate of soda (baking soda) to the warm water and soak for at least 15 minutes. This gentle solution also acts as a deodorizer and soother for over-exerted feet. Remove and towel-dry lightly so that the feet are not soaking wet when you begin the scrubbing treatment.

2 Smooth away problem areas with a foot file or pumice stone. Work over the heels, sides and soles of your feet, but do not treat the toes with it as the skin here is softer, and may blister. A loofah or body scrubber is a good alternative to using a pumice stone. Remember that if the foot begins to feel tender, you should finish this stage of the treatment and move on to the next. A build-up of hard skin should be removed gradually; you can scrub the feet again in a day or so.

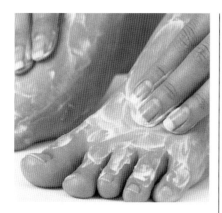

3 You should apply foot cream to your feet on a daily basis – as regularly as you moisturize the other areas of your body. Rub the cream in well, avoiding moisture-prone spaces between the toes where bacteria can grow. Once a week, apply an extra thick layer of cream to your feet, allowing the skin to absorb it, and then put on a pair of thin cotton socks to hold in the moisture overnight. Your feet will be noticeably softer in the morning for this replenishing treatment.

treating the ankles

The ankles and shins are as susceptible to dry, flaky skin as the feet are to calluses. The following treatment uses a light, feathery touch, similar to a massage technique, to remove dead skin cells and stimulate circulation.

Blend 2 drops of essential oil, such as mandarin, with 20ml / 4 tsp of carrier oil. Dampen a soft-bristled brush with warm water. Then pour about 5ml / 1 tsp of the oil over the bristles. Gently rub the brush over the top of the foot, using upward strokes. Rub up the heel and around the ankle area, followed by the front, and then the back, of the lower leg, all the while using upward strokes. Cover this whole area a total of three times, adding more oil as necessary.

Wipe off any excess oil with a cloth. Then use the same cloth to stroke gently all over the top of the foot and the front of the lower leg, until the area feels completely dry and comfortable.

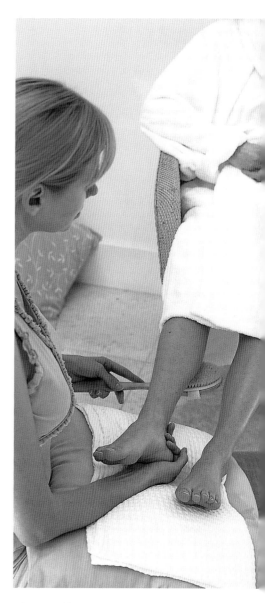

above *Ankles and feet will benefit from this regular exfoliation routine.*

essential stress-relievers

Stress is often held in the digestive and respiratory systems. This set of reflexology moves aims to remove tension in these areas, so that the organs can function well.

During stress, the "fight or flight" syndrome prompts the release of the hormone adrenaline, which impacts the body in many ways. Symptoms include a racing heart, tension headaches, shortness of breath, neck aches and high blood pressure. Stress can take years off your life, so learning to control it will improve overall health.

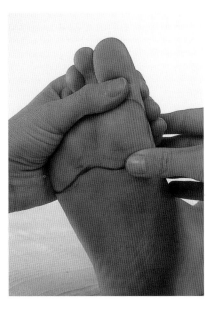

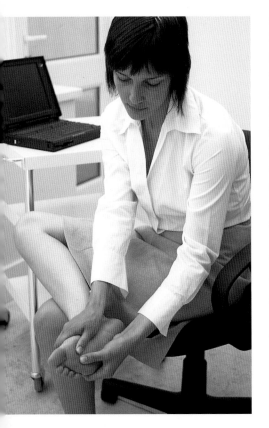

neutralizing stress

It is essential to organize your day so that you take regular breaks – even just two 10-minute breaks, in the morning and afternoon, can help prevent stress build-up. Regular exercise, especially in the fresh air, helps burn pent-up energy that would otherwise overload the system. Exercise also aids sound sleep, which is very important – the body needs this time to recuperate from daily activity and ward off possible infection.

Reflexology can help combat stress by targeting specific areas of the body that may be holding tension. While you are learning these techniques, it may be useful to draw the zones you wish to treat on the feet using an eyebrow pencil, as shown in these exercises.

left *Reflexology may be practised at work or home to reduce stress build-up.*

1 To relax the diaphragm, hold the foot as shown, lowering it on to the thumb of your other hand and then lifting it off again. Now move your thumb one step towards the outer side of the foot, gradually working to the outer edge and back again until you have thumb-walked across the boundary line of the ball of the foot. By relieving tightness in the diaphragm, the muscle works more freely.

The four exercises below can be performed alone or with a partner. For best results, work on bare feet — but if it's impractical to remove tights or socks, you will still be able to apply the kind of pressure needed to stimulate energy flow.

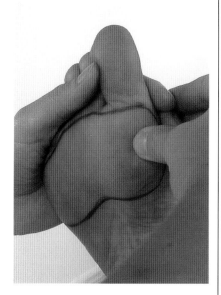

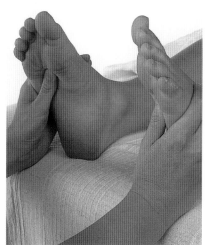

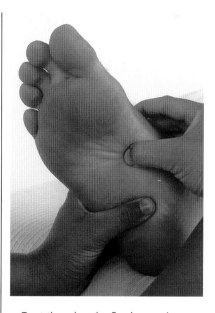

2 Now the diaphragm is relaxed, you are free to work the lung reflexes on the chest area, which is slightly higher up the foot. Use the same thumb-walking motion to cover the reflexes of this zone. You will find that your breathing becomes deeper, drawing more air into your lungs. As the blood takes in more oxygen, you will feel the symptoms of anxiety begin to subside.

3 This solar plexus breathing exercise can be done by working on both feet at the same time. Hold each foot, positioning your thumbs in the centre of the diaphragm line. As you breathe in, gently press in with your thumbs, holding for a couple of seconds, and release again as you breathe out. Repeat several times, until you find a natural rhythm in your breathing.

4 Treat the adrenal reflex by rotating gently on the thumb in the position shown. This will ease the release of adrenaline, the hormone that triggers the "fight or flight" syndrome. By reducing the amount of adrenaline, stress symptoms such as raised blood pressure, tension headaches and obstructed digestion should start to decrease, allowing your body to function more efficiently again.

post-workout pummelling

Use this set of exercises to soothe and calm muscles that have worked hard during exercise.
If at home, soaking the feet in a foot bath is a useful prelude to treatment.

Make sure the feet are thoroughly dry before beginning. If desired, use a small
amount of massage oil and rub between the palms to warm.

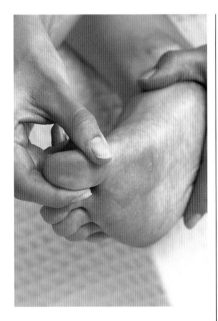

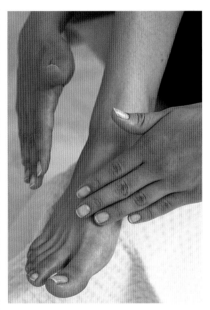

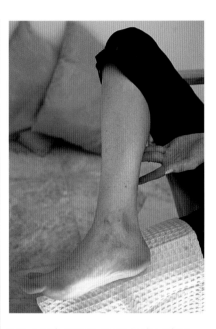

1 Start with the right foot. Use the thumb
and index finger of your left hand to
pull your big toe straight, and hold to
a count of five. Gently rotate it in a
clockwise direction, then repeat with an
anticlockwise movement. Do the same
for all the other toes, then move on to
the left foot.

2 Once again, begin with the right foot,
making sure that it is supported by a
soft, cushioned surface. Use the tips of
the fingers to slap all over the foot,
including the sole, sides and ankle.
Make the slaps as heavy as you can,
but lighter on the top of the foot. This
technique helps to break down toxins.

3 To guard against cramp in the calves,
put two fingers across the Achilles
tendon, then slide upwards until you
feel the taut base of the calf muscle.
Press into this part of the muscle and
make deep circular movements. Work
in this way up the leg, treating the
entire muscle. Repeat several times.

right The soles of the feet are prone to dryness and cracking, especially after the impact of exercise. It is well worth massaging them with oil at least once a week, to ensure that they remain soft, supple and sufficiently moisturized.

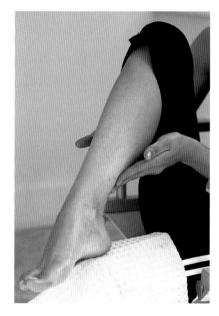

4 Finish off with some gentle relaxation work. Placing the hands close together, so they jut out in opposite directions, briskly stroke up the back of the leg, covering the area from the ankle to the knee. Slide the hands back down to the ankle and repeat twice.

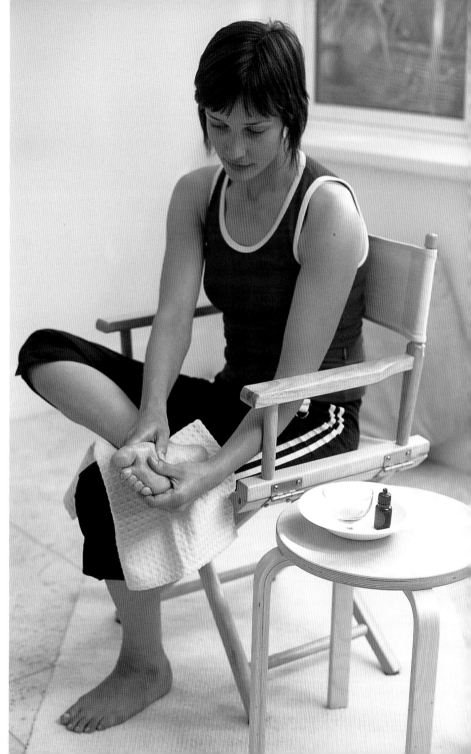

immunity-boosting acupressure

Acupressure involves pressing or lightly pinching points on the feet to direct a flow of healing energy to the organs. Each organ may correspond to several points on the foot.

Start this self-treatment by massaging the feet gently to relax them, and make them receptive to energy flow. **Caution:** Avoid during the first trimester of pregnancy.

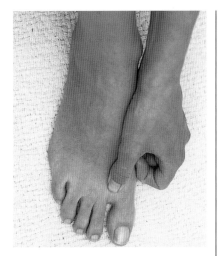

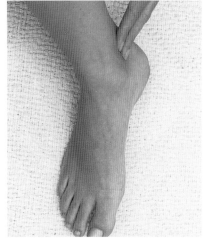

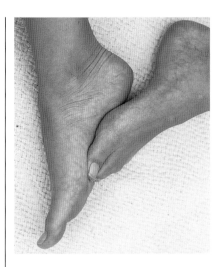

1 Put your right foot flat on the floor, and place your thumb in the groove between the big and second toes. Slide the thumb up this groove, then back down towards the base of the toes. Repeat twice, applying firm pressure. This works acupressure point Liver 3, which helps to counter the symptoms of stress.

2 Place your index and middle fingers between the inner ankle bone and the slight bulge formed by the Achilles tendon. Press for a count of 20, then release for a count of 30. Repeat twice. This works Kidney 3, which is good for boosting energy levels following a period of intense work, which may have left you drained.

3 Repeat steps 1 and 2 on the left foot. Now turn the right foot on its side so that the inner edge points upwards. Use the toes of the left foot to massage along the edge, working from heel to toe. Repeat for the left foot. This works the liver and spleen, aiding the production of natural antibodies to fight infection.

right *During dance and exercise, you may be stimulating many acupressure points at once, giving your immune system a real boost.*

The following two acupressure points are located in the ankle area and shins. Remember to pay equal attention to both legs, beginning with the right.

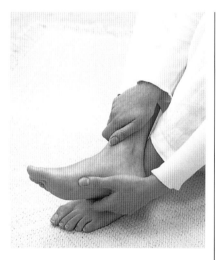

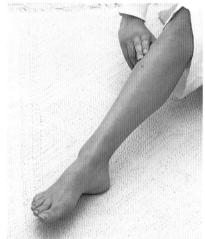

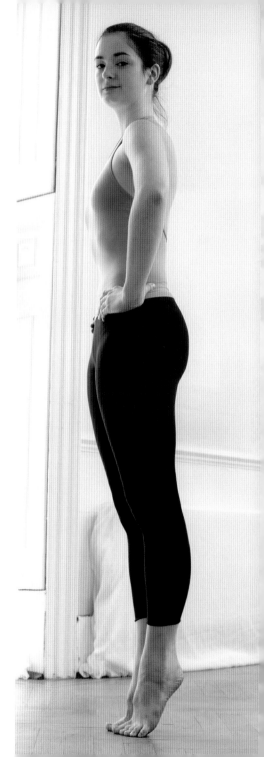

1 Put the thumb of your left hand on the inner side of the right foot, about one thumb-width below the ball. Press and hold for 30 seconds, breathing deeply. Release the point slowly, breathe for a count of 20, then press again for another 30 seconds. Do the left foot in the same way. This exercise works Spleen 4, which helps to fight off a cold.

2 Place the two middle fingers of your right hand on the outside of the right lower leg. The fingers should be four finger-widths down from the kneecap and one finger-width towards the outside of the shinbone. This point is Stomach 36, which is used for a quick energy boost. Rub up and down to the count of 50, breathing as you work. Rest for a minute, then repeat.

beautifying pedicure

Regular foot care should always include treatment of the toenails. A weekly pedicure will keep the feet looking attractive and healthy all through the year.

First, create a pedicurist's essential kit, to include nail clippers, cotton buds, an emery board, toe separators or cotton wool, clear or coloured nail polish and polish remover.

1 Trim the toenails using nail clippers or specially curved scissors, working straight across the nail. Using an emery board, file your toenails straight across, rounding them slightly at the corners. Do not file into the corners or you will encourage the formation of painful in-grown toenails.

2 Next, rub cuticle cream into the base of the nails; alternatively, you could use almond or olive oil. Massage the cream or oil into the nails and cuticles, one at a time, using circular movements. This not only prepares the cuticles for shaping, it protects and nourishes the nails as well.

3 Allow a few minutes for the cream or oil to soften the cuticles. Now gently push back each cuticle with a hoof stick or cotton bud, using quick, light movements – don't try to force tough cuticles all at once. Next, wipe off traces of cream thoroughly and finish with a coat of clear nail strengthener.

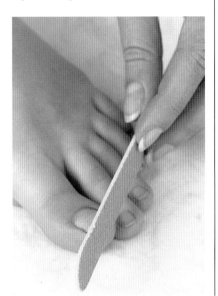
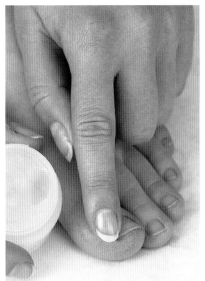
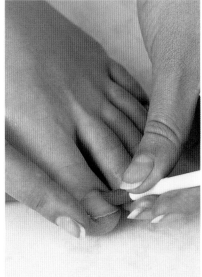

applying nail polish

Generally, the toes will take much brighter colours than the fingers, so you can experiment with bright, funky hues. However, if you don't wish to draw too much attention to your feet, choose classic clear polish or neutral pinks.

1 If you like, you can separate your toes with either cotton wool or a foam rubber toe separator. Alternatively, you can weave a twisted tissue between your toes if neither of the above are handy. Apply a base coat of clear nail polish to create a smooth surface on which to work. This will also prevent brightly coloured polishes from permanently staining the nails.

2 With the chosen polish, work each nail by painting a stripe of colour down the middle, then overlap with a strip of colour down each side. Leave to dry thoroughly, then apply another coat. Finish with a clear top coat to make the polish extra hard-wearing, and wait for one hour before putting on socks, tights or shoes, so that the polish is properly sealed.

right *Pedicures are easy to do at home and you can create your own look.*

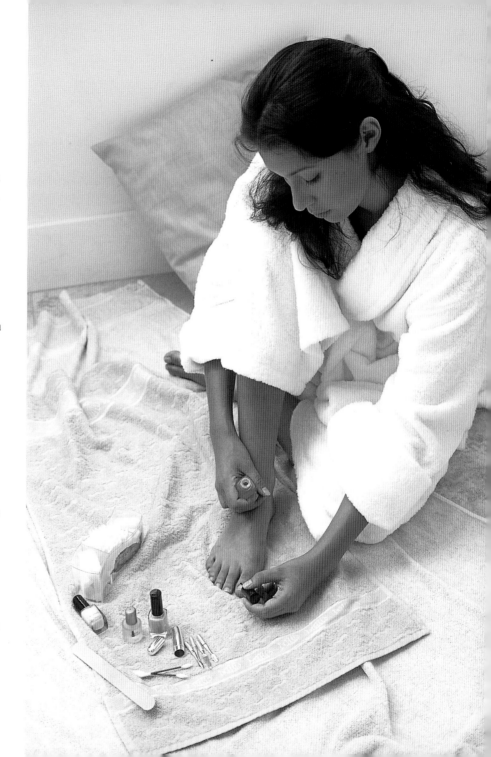

calming bedtime massage

Our feet are in constant use throughout the day and a little night-time TLC will help to relax them, inducing sleepiness. Perform this massage with your partner at bedtime.

Prepare a fragrant night-time massage oil by blending a few drops of bergamot, neroli or sandalwood essential oil with a carrier. These oils promote feelings of calm.

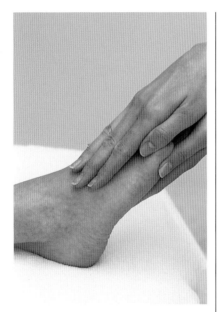 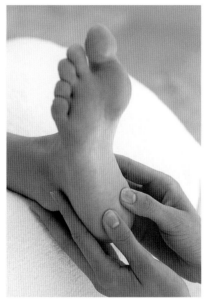 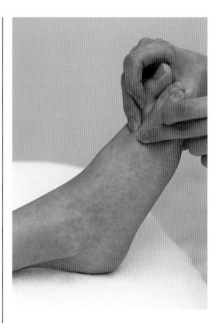

1 Hold the right foot in a "sandwich" with your hands – place one hand lengthways over the top of the foot, the other underneath it. Slide the hands up the foot to the toes and back again. Repeat several times, increasing the pressure as you go.

2 Now place your thumbs on the heel, one slightly higher than the other. Massage by rotating in tiny circles with your thumbs. Work up the foot, using lighter pressure on the arch – a sensitive area, prone to discomfort – than on the heel and ball.

3 Massage the top of the foot in the same way, but use your two middle fingers. Start in the groove between the big and second toe, and work down the foot to the ankle. Repeat, starting between the second and third toes. Work across the foot in the same way.

right *Massage at bedtime is not only soothing and relaxing, it is also a sensual experience, perfect for sharing with your partner. You will both benefit from this time together, and the mutual bond established by therapeutic touch.*

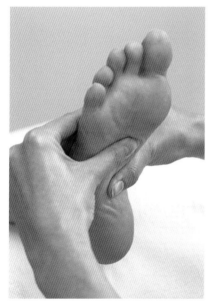

4 Place your thumbs on the sole pointing in opposite directions. Slide the thumbs up the sole, making a criss-cross movement, so that the left thumb goes under the right, then right above left. From the toes, work down the foot then back up again. Repeat on the left foot.

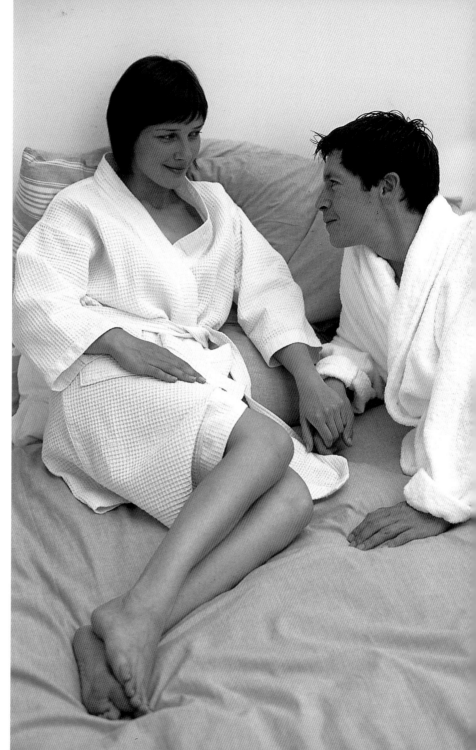

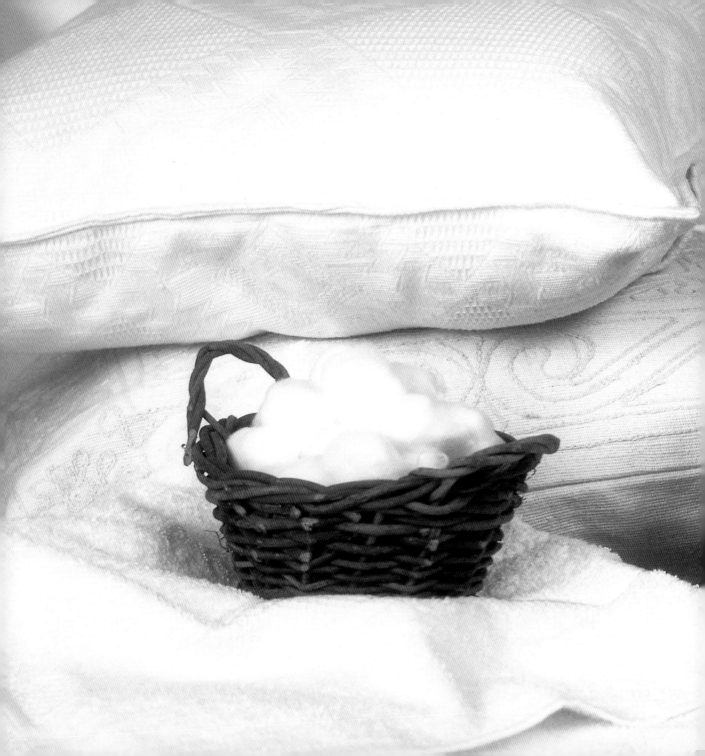

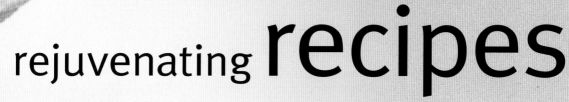

rejuvenating recipes

By using just a few simple, pure-quality ingredients, you can make your own pampering and nourishing potions. These revitalizing and fragrant scrubs, oils, baths and lotions will give your feet an uplifting treat at the end of the day.

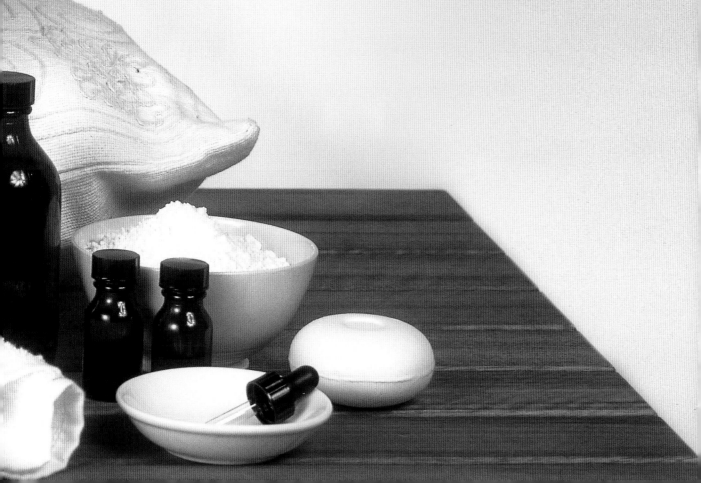

botanical foot baths

A foot bath is an easy and effective way to refresh tired feet. As well as warming and relaxing aching muscles and joints, the vapours in these herbal baths calm the mind.

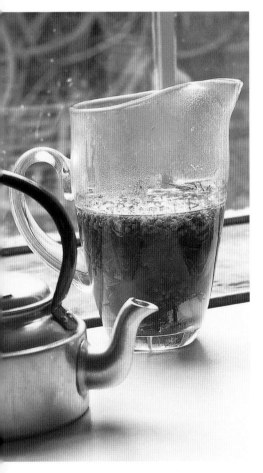

above *Steeped fresh herbs stimulate the senses as well as soothing the body.*

These simple recipes call for either dried or fresh herbs infused in hot water. Plants all have different beneficial properties: pine needles and peppermint oil stimulate the tissues and ease aches and pains, while lavender helps rejuvenate the cells and chamomile has a calming effect on the nerves.

herbal foot bath for aching feet

The fresh herbs included here can be found in many gardens and fields, but you can substitute dried herbs if some are difficult to get hold of. The Epsom salts and borax that are added to this foot bath give it extra soothing and purifying qualities.

50g / 2oz mixed fresh herbs such as peppermint, yarrow, pine needles, chamomile flowers, rosemary, houseleek
1 litre / 1³/₄ pints / 4 cups boiling water
15ml / 1 tbsp borax
15ml / 1 tbsp Epsom salts

1 Roughly chop the herbs, put them in a large bowl and pour in the boiling water. Leave to stand for one hour.
2 Strain the herbs, then add to a bowl containing about 1.75 litres / 3 pints / 7¹/₂ cups hot water – the temperature of the foot bath should be comfortably warm, but not so hot as to scald.
3 Stir in the borax and Epsom salts, immerse the feet and soak for 15–20 minutes.

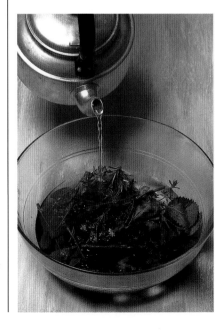

lemon verbena and lavender foot bath

This aromatic bath combines the gentle cleansing properties of lavender with the zesty aroma of lemon verbena to wake up the whole body while regenerating the feet. Cider vinegar is recognized as a useful conditioner for the hair and skin.

30ml / 2 tbsp dried lavender or crushed
   fresh lavender
15g / ¹/₂oz dried lemon verbena
5 drops lavender essential oil
30ml / 2 tbsp cider vinegar

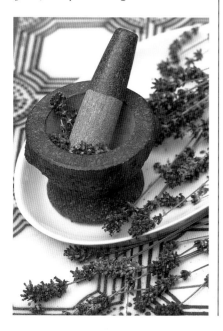

1 If you have gathered fresh lavender flowers, make sure they are rinsed thoroughly, and then crush using a pestle and mortar to release the natural perfume and oils. You can use dried herbs to save a little time on preparation, if you wish.
2 Place the lemon verbena and lavender in a bowl and pour in enough boiling water to cover the feet. When it has cooled to a comfortable temperature, add the lavender oil and cider vinegar and soak the feet for 20 minutes to repair and condition the skin tissues.

lavender essential oil

This cold-infused oil is a useful addition to many bath and massage oils. You can prepare your own lavender oil in just a few simple steps.

1 First, fill a glass storage jar with the cleaned flowers or leaves of the plant.
2 Pour in a light vegetable oil to cover the plant matter – try sunflower or grapeseed oil. Seal tightly.
3 Allow the oil to stand on a windowsill for a month, to allow the essential oil and aroma to permeate the liquid. Shake the jar gently every day.
4 Strain the ingredients, pour the oil into dark bottles and keep for eight weeks.

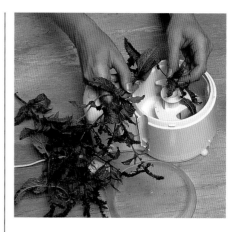

mint foot bath

Fresh mint is an excellent tonic for sore feet, and has a soothing aroma.

12 large sprigs of mint
120ml / 4fl oz / ¹/₂ cup cold water
2.5 litres / 4 pints / 10 cups boiling water
15ml / 1 tbsp almond oil
1 drop mint essential oil

1 Place the sprigs of mint and cold water in a food processor, and purée to a green paste.
2 Place the purée in a large bowl with the boiling water. Allow to cool to bearable heat, and soak the feet.
3 After soaking, gently towel-dry the feet and combine the almond oil and mint essential oil. Rub well into both feet.

smoothing foot scrubs

Instead of using a loofah for exfoliating the feet and ankles, you can try a heady-scented scrub to remove rough, flaky skin and smooth the outer layers of the epidermis.

Each of the following foot scrubs should be applied after a warm bath, when the feet are damp but not soaking wet. Both recipes make around 150g / 5oz, so store any leftovers in a glass container, and use within two weeks.

orange and almond foot scrub

This citrus scrub is perfect for feet. The grittiness of the ground oatmeal and almonds helps rid the skin of impurities and dead cells, while the orange rind and rose petals stimulate and tone the skin. Essential oils work to feed and moisturize this often neglected part of the body.

30ml / 2 tbsp powdered orange rind
45ml / 3 tbsp ground almonds
30ml / 2 tbsp oatmeal
15ml / 1 tbsp rose petals
90ml / 6 tbsp almond oil
5 drops flower essential oil, such as rose, jasmine or neroli
5 drops wood essential oil, such as sandalwood or cedar

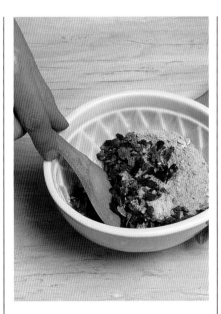

1 Mix all the dry ingredients together in a bowl, taking care to combine thoroughly. Powdered orange rind is a useful, ready-prepared confectionery item, but freshly grated orange or lemon peel will also do. Add the almond oil one tablespoon at a time, and blend in gradually with the other ingredients, until the mixture becomes a crumbly paste.

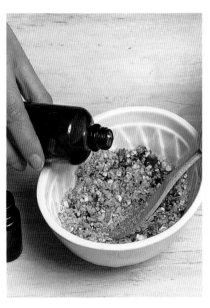

2 Stir in your chosen essential oils and blend completely. After soaking both feet and towel-drying thoroughly, take a handful of the mixture and rub it into your skin, one foot at a time, paying particular attention to the areas of dry, rough skin on the edges of the feet and the ankles. Leave the scrub to dry on the skin, and then remove, gently, using a dry flannel.

jojoba and glycerine foot scrub

This exfoliating scrub can be used when your feet need a bit of a boost. Glycerine has a nourishing effect, while the fuller's earth and salt help to deep-cleanse.

10ml / 2 tsp foaming foot or bath wash
2 drops mandarin and 1 drop geranium
   essential oils (or substitute with lavender
   and lemon oils if not available)
5 ml / 1 tsp glycerine
5 ml / 1 tsp each fuller's earth & rock salt
5ml / 1 tsp almond oil
5ml / 1 tsp jojoba oil

1 In a small clean bottle, combine the foaming wash, essential oils and glycerine. Shake and set aside while you prepare the other ingredients.

2 Put the fuller's earth and rock salt into a medium-sized bowl and mix together well. Add the almond and jojoba oils, and again combine thoroughly.

3 Add the glycerine mixture to the bowl and mix all the ingredients together with a metal spoon. You should now have a runny paste, which can be easily applied to the feet.

right Set out all the ingredients in clean bowls and bottles before beginning.

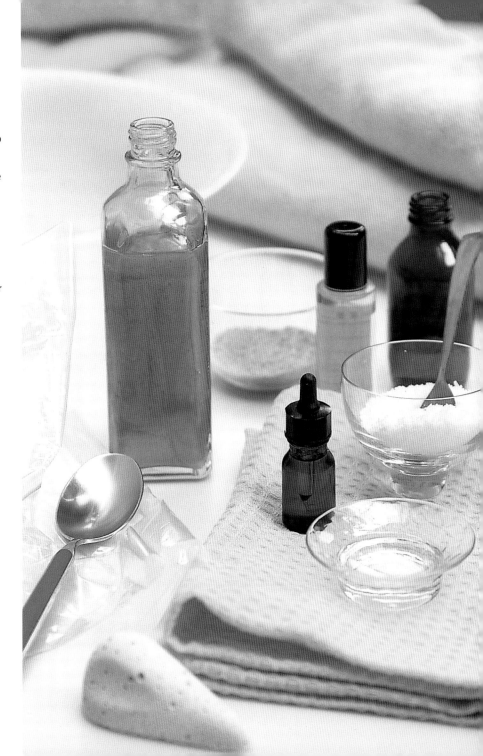

stimulating aromatherapy oils

After a bath, you can treat aching or tired feet to a rejuvenating aromatherapy massage. These recipes are simple and easy to make, and store well for future use.

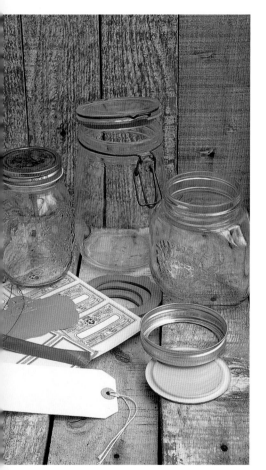

above Oils are best stored in glass jars, away from light and heat.

To make any of the following recipes, simply pour the ingredients into a sterile glass bottle or jar with a stopper and shake to blend. All make about 50ml / 2fl oz.

aching muscle reliever

This blend brings quick relief to feet suffering tension and stiffness due to over-exertion from jogging, sport or standing for prolonged periods. Pine oil works to relieve fatigue, while rosemary oil helps to stimulate circulation and ease fluid retention.

45ml / 3 tbsp carrier oil such as grapeseed or almond
10 drops rosemary essential oil
10 drops pine essential oil

1 To apply, take a small amount of the oil blend into your hands, and rub together to warm thoroughly.
2 Now work the oil into the foot, ankle and calf area using the palms of your hands. Massage vigorously: this boosts the circulation and enables a faster absorption of the essential oils. Swap to work on the other foot and repeat the whole process.

circulation improver

This massage oil uses essential oil of black pepper, which has properties that stimulate the circulation and help to warm the tissues. If your circulation is poor, the first sign is cold extremities – your fingers and toes may become numb and sometimes the toes may turn blue due to lack of blood supply.

45ml / 3 tbsp carrier oil such as grapeseed or almond
10 drops black pepper essential oil

1 If your toes are very cold, massage them to warm before treating with oil.
2 Next, take a small amount of oil blend and rub between your hands. Massage into the top and sides of the foot, and work well into the dry spots on the arch and sole. Spread the oil down to the toes, lightly massaging each one in turn, right down to the tips. Repeat with the other foot.

cooling refresher

Perfect for use on hot, aching feet, this massage blend cools and refreshes the skin and sinks deep into the tissues. Peppermint oil is widely used in herbal remedies – it contains menthol, which is known for its cooling and antispasmodic properties. Light and refreshing, lemon oil has cleansing, antiseptic properties.

45ml / 3 tbsp carrier oil, such as
grapeseed or almond
10 drops peppermint essential oil
10 drops lemon essential oil

Massaging with this deodorizing blend gives your feet a well-deserved treat after a long walk or run in hiking shoes or trainers. You can also use it as an after-work pick-me-up, when your feet have been trapped in shoes all day. The gentle aromas of mint and lemon will give the whole body a gentle lift, too, and help to dissolve fatigue.

right *Aromatherapy oils are most effective when massaged into cleansed feet, directly after a shower or foot bath. A simple spreading movement, using the pads of the thumbs to rub in the oils, will aid their absorption by the skin.*

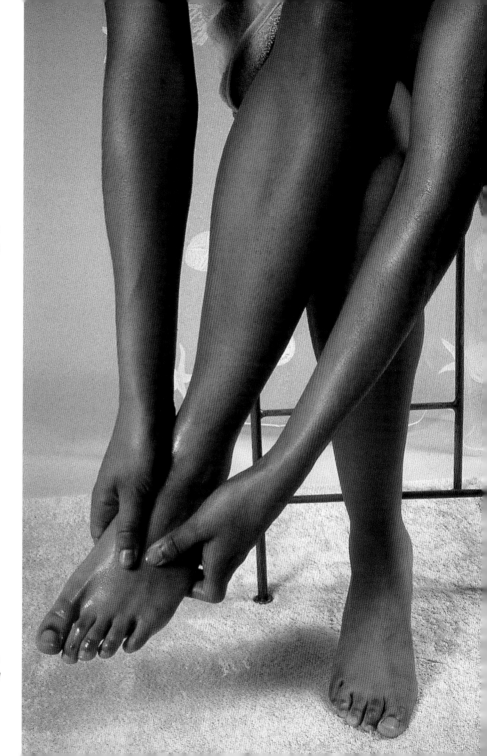

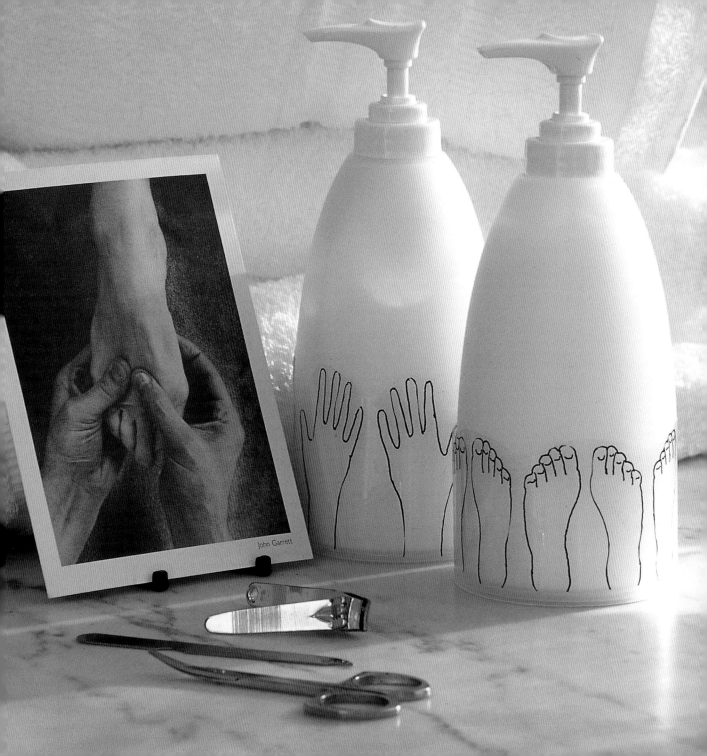

John Garrett

herbal foot creams

It is easy to make rich, heady-scented creams to moisturize the rough skin on feet. Look out for lanolin-rich or Vitamin E creams as a base, as these help to repair the skin.

These foot creams are very quick to prepare: simply add essential oils to an unscented pot of purchased cream. Store in a plastic pump-action bottle, or a tightly-lidded glass jar or ceramic pot. Both recipes make around 120ml / 4fl oz.

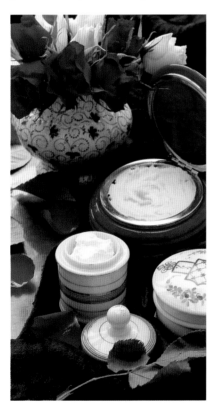

left *Store your herbal creams in pretty jars or handy pump bottles.*

floral foot cream

Essential oils in this cream nourish the feet: chamomile soothes, geranium helps heal cuts and lemon oil softens the skin. The emollient properties of Vitamin E cream make this a good overnight moisturizer for very dry, rough skin.

120ml / 4fl oz / ½ cup unscented hand cream, preferably rich in Vitamin E or jojoba oil
7 drops chamomile essential oil
7 drops geranium essential oil
7 drops lemon essential oil

1 Place the unscented hand cream in a small bowl and blend in the essential oils thoroughly. You may find it easier to use a whisk to ensure that the ingredients combine properly.
2 Pour into a clean, pump-action bottle using a funnel. Simply apply to feet and allow to absorb.

tea tree and lemon foot cream

The active ingredient in this recipe is tea tree oil, which has an antiseptic and antifungal action. This cream is a cooling and refreshing moisturizer for hot, tired, hard-working feet.

120ml / 4fl oz / ½ cup unscented hand cream, preferably Vitamin E or jojoba
12 drops tea tree essential oil
7 drops lemon essential oil

Follow the instructions for preparation as for the Floral Foot Cream. Wearing a pair of thin cotton socks, once the cream has been absorbed by the skin, will maximize its nourishing effects.

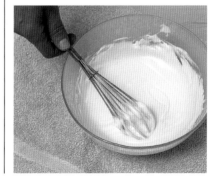

soothing foot powders

Dusting powder is a soothing, cooling way to keep feet dry and help prevent perspiration. These preparations boast delicious fragrances for all-day freshness.

Powders add a wonderful finishing flourish to your home spa experience. Easy to blend at home, you can adapt the ingredients according to preference.

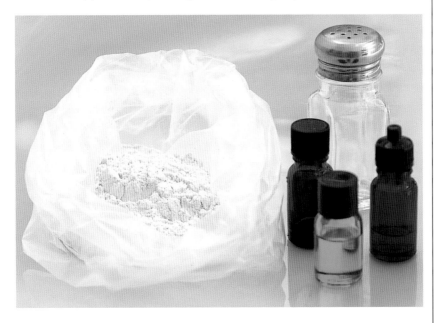

1 Mix together the rice flour, orris root and bicarbonate of soda. Add the teaspoon of boric acid powder and mix well.

2 Drop in the essential oils and stir until absorbed. Transfer the powder to a clean plastic shaker.

below Strongly antiseptic, antibacterial and antifungal, essential oil from the tea tree plant is often used with a carrier, but can also be applied, undiluted, to treat athlete's foot and verrucas.

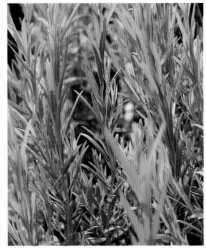

cooling sport powder

This is a wonderful powder to use before and after playing sport or dancing. Tea tree is an essential component because of its antiseptic qualities, but you could swap the lemon oil for other fragrant oils such as sandalwood or rosemary. This recipe makes around 175g / 6oz.

50g / 2oz rice flour

50g / 2oz orris root powder

50g / 2oz bicarbonate of soda (baking soda)

5ml / 1 tsp boric acid powder

6 drops tea tree essential oil

6 drops lemon essential oil

sumptuous rose powder

This is a heavenly scented powder that uses rose essential oil and either mica silk – a powdered mineral – or unscented talcum powder as its base. The proportions below make around 175g / 6oz, but you can prepare more or less, simply by using the ratio of 5 parts powder to 1 part cornflour. Store in a glass jar with a tightly-fitted lid, so that moisture cannot penetrate.

150g / 5oz mica silk or talcum powder
25g / 1oz cornflour (cornstarch)
9 drops rose essential oil

1 Mix the dry ingredients thoroughly.
2 Add the rose oil gradually, and stir in until absorbed completely and powder is dry in consistency. Apply to the feet with powder puff or hands.

Rose is a classic scent that lifts the spirits and calms the nerves. However, instead of using rose oil you could substitute your favourite floral essence, such as jasmine, geranium or melissa.

right *Dusting with a perfumed powder helps keep your feet dry all day, and its bouquet lingers to boost your mood.*

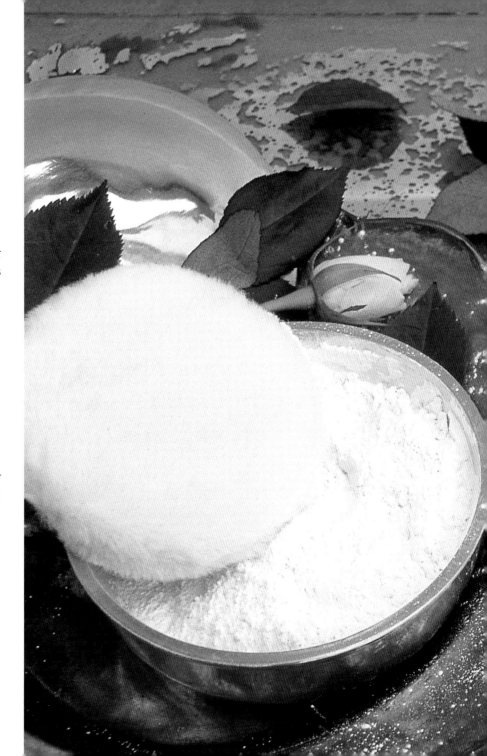

nourishing masks

When used on the feet, moisturizing and polishing masks combat rough skin and cracks on the soles and heels due to sun exposure or friction.

Masks can help improve the texture of the skin, tightening it and helping to reduce the occurrence of lines. As these recipes contain fresh ingredients, make each on the day that you plan to use it, and do not store leftovers. Apply the mask to the feet and leave on for 15 minutes. Rinse off and follow with a moisturizing oil or cream.

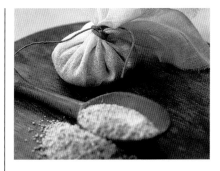

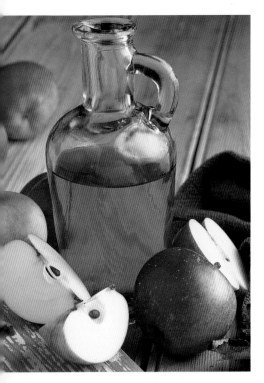

above *Fresh mask ingredients, good enough to eat, ensure pure skincare.*

apple and honey foot mask

This mask will tone and moisturize dry skin, and its delicious, clean aroma will delight the senses. Fresh apple contains active enzymes to revitalize the skin, and egg yolk provides a cocktail of vitamins and minerals to nourish it. The antibacterial attributes of honey make it a useful addition to skin treatments.

1 egg yolk
1 small apple, peeled and grated
15ml / 1 tbsp honey
45ml / 3 tbsp almond oil

Beat the egg yolk lightly and then blend with the apple and honey. Add the almond oil a little at a time to make a thick paste – depending on the juiciness of the apple, you may need a little more or less than 45ml to produce the correct consistency.

oatmeal foot mask

Finely ground almonds or powdered rind will provide the gritty base to this mask. Use yogurt to blend the dry ingredients if your skin tends to be oily, or replace this with almond oil if you have dry skin.

10ml / 2 tsp fine oatmeal
30ml / 2 tbsp powdered orange rind
  (or 30ml / 2 tbsp finely ground almonds)
yogurt or almond oil, to blend

Mix the dry ingredients together and add enough yogurt or almond oil to make a thick paste.

right *Be sure to rub a little oil or cream into the feet after rinsing away the mask.*

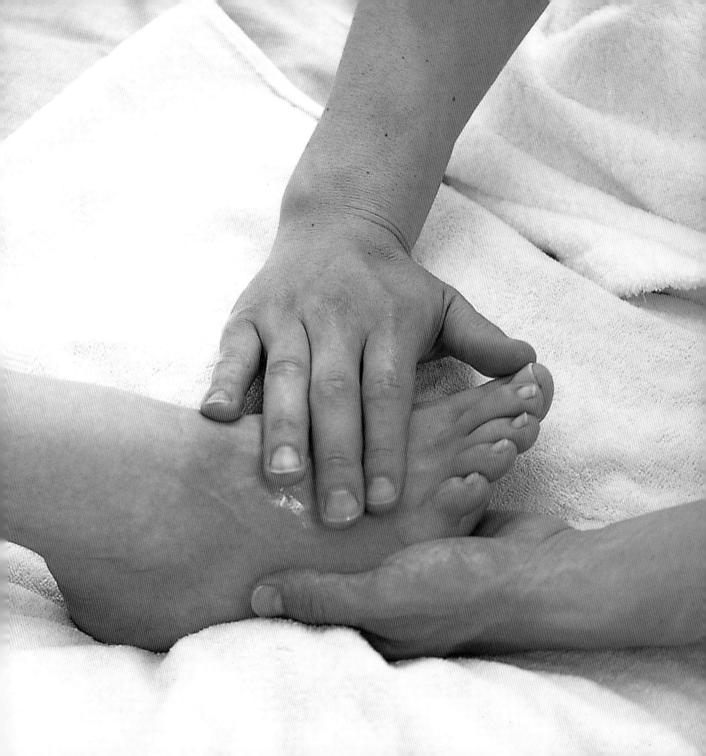

antibacterial boosters

Active feet may become prone to fungal infections when tight shoes – especially trainers
– are worn for extended periods. Antifungal herbs can help to ease the discomfort.

A fungal condition caused by dermatophytes (parasites on the skin), known as athlete's foot, can cause an uncomfortable, itchy red rash and burning sensations in the feet. This contagious fungus can be picked up via skin contact, or from infected towels, locker room floors, socks and shoes.

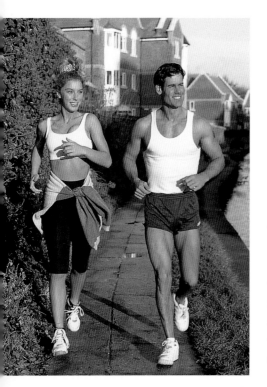

above *Following a foot hygiene routine is important if you jog or walk regularly.*

antifungal foot bath

This foot bath is suitable for soothing athlete's foot. The cider vinegar helps to restore pH balance of the skin, which becomes over-alkaline when this condition is present. Myrrh (a resin) and tea tree oil both have antifungal properties, and aloe vera is a highly beneficial succulent that is used worldwide to accelerate the healing of many skin conditions, and is also used to treat burns, cuts and bruises.

Make the foot bath fresh each time.

1 large aloe vera leaf, chopped
25g / 1oz dried lavender
25g / 1oz dried pot marigold flowers
15ml / 1 tbsp myrrh granules
2.5 litres / 4 pints / 10 cups
   boiling water
10 drops tea tree essential oil
60ml / 4 tbsp cider vinegar

1 Steep the herbs and myrrh together in the boiling water for 20 minutes. Leave to cool a little, then strain using muslin (cheesecloth) as shown. Reheat gently until hand-hot.

2 Add the tea tree oil and cider vinegar.

3 Pour the hand-hot mixture into a foot bath and immerse the feet for up to 15 minutes. After bathing, you can ensure dryness by sprinkling the feet with a talc or antifungal powder. Always wear cotton or wool socks, and change them twice daily

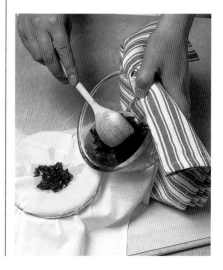

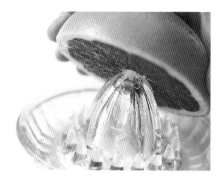

sage and grapefruit foot bath

With their antibacterial properties, fresh sage leaves make this a good preventive treatment for infection. A powerful cleanser with an uplifting scent, grapefruit also acts to open the pores.

25g / 1oz fresh sage leaves
2.5 litres / 4 pints / 10 cups water
1 grapefruit, juiced, or 10 drops
    grapefruit essential oil

1 Simmer the sage leaves in water for 20 minutes. Leave to cool, then strain through muslin (cheesecloth).
2 Pour the mixture into a bowl and add the grapefruit juice or essential oil; swirl to blend. Apply to cleansed feet.

right *Always allow feet to dry thoroughly to help prevent infection and fungus.*

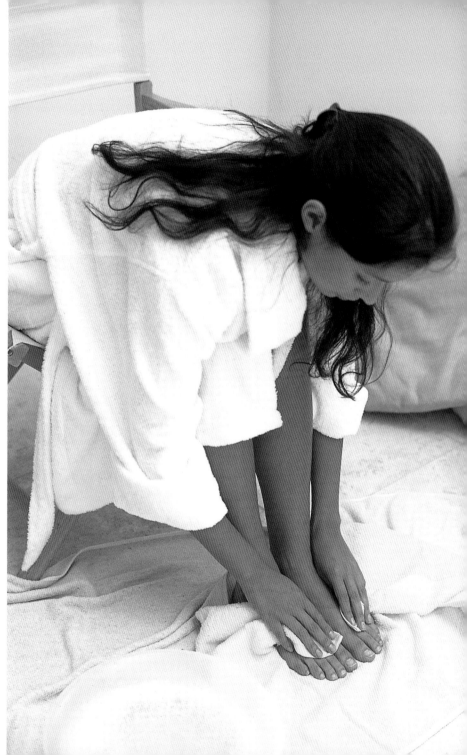

hypertension reliever

As part of an after-work pampering treatment, these relaxing foot baths help reduce heightened stress levels that can cause temporary hypertension, or ease a pre-existing condition.

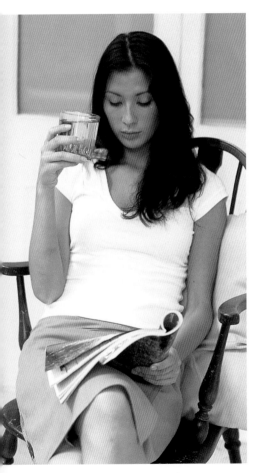

above *Taking time to relax may lower blood pressure and add years to your life.*

High blood pressure often shows no symptoms and goes undetected, so routine medical check-ups are important. If diagnosed, treatments may vary from patient to patient, and should be discussed with your doctor. In some cases of hypertension, especially those brought on by stress, essential oils are said to lower elevated levels.

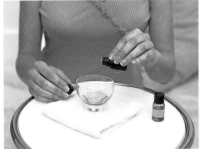

melissa and lavender foot bath

Melissa is said to quell anxiety and calm nerves, lowering the blood pressure.

3 drops melissa essential oil
3 drops lavender essential oil
3 drops ylang ylang essential oil

1 Fill a large bowl three-quarters full with hand-hot water.
2 Blend the essential oils together and add to the water a few drops at a time, swirling to disperse. Soak the feet for at least 10 minutes.

making time to relax

After you've soaked your feet, it is worth indulging in a little aftercare for the whole body, simply by giving yourself the time to relax.

Towel-dry your feet thoroughly and find a quiet place to rest for about half an hour. Simply close your eyes and meditate or daydream, listen to some soothing music or read a book. There are many relaxation CDs and tapes available with exercises that can help you control anxious feelings, so that you can put your life into perspective.

By choosing to minimize the stress in your life, and by resolving to take control of your emotions and your reactions to people and situations, you will go a long way towards keeping body and mind in good health. This new clarity of thought will enable you to act decisively, and to focus on what really matters to you.

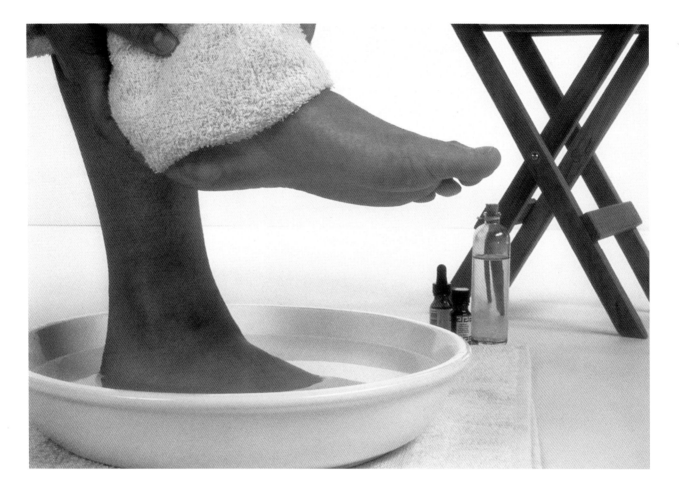

clary sage compress

This compress contains clary sage, which may help in lowering blood pressure, and petitgrain, which may ease swollen ankles caused by water retention. You can use a small hand towel or tea cloth for the compress. Be sure to relax during treatment to reap maximum benefit.

300ml / ½ pint / 1¼ cups hand-hot water

2 drops clary sage essential oil

2 drops petitgrain essential oil

1 Put the hand-hot water into a sink or large bowl.

2 Add the drops of essential oil and swirl to disperse.

3 Dampen a towel or cloth with the blend and wrap around the feet. Sit back and relax for 10 to 15 minutes.

Caution: Clary sage should not be used during the first three months of pregnancy. Do not use with alcohol. In larger doses, it may cause headaches.

rich lavender moisturizer

Feet are overworked and under-moisturized, and soles and heels are often left crying
out with thirst. This rich oil will help keep the skin healthy, soft and callus-free.

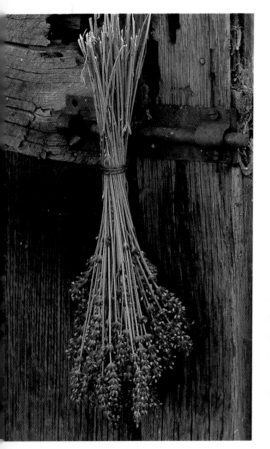

above *Lavender oil is an ideal addition
to moisturizers, thanks to its soothing
fragrance and skin-healing properties.*

Lubricating the feet is important, especially during extremes of temperature. The cold, harsh conditions of winter can redden the skin, causing irritated, itchy feet. In the summer months, wearing sandals exposes your feet to hot sun, dust, sand and dirt – not to mention chlorine from swimming pools – leaving skin parched and cracked.

lavender moisturizer

This fragrant moisturizer combines the emollient properties of pure almond oil with the cell-rejuvenating effects of lavender. Chamomile oil is added to calm and soothe dry skin. This recipe makes around 50ml / 2fl oz, and any excess can be stored in a glass bottle with stopper. Use on damp skin while pores are open.

45ml / 3 tbsp almond oil
1.5ml / $^{1}/_{4}$ tsp wheatgerm oil
15 drops lavender essential oil
5 drops chamomile essential oil

1 Pour the almond and wheatgerm oils into a glass bottle, add the essential oils and gently shake to mix. Store the bottle in a cool, dark place. In the summer months, you may want to refrigerate the blend, which will give your skin a cooling treat.

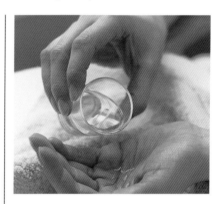

2 To apply, place a small amount of oil in the palms and rub to warm. Work into feet and legs, massaging gently until the lotion has been completely absorbed. You can use it as a body moisturizer too – just continue massaging upwards to your torso, neck and finally, your arms and hands.

right *Protect the feet from cracking with regular moisturizing. You can combine with massage for a real treat.*

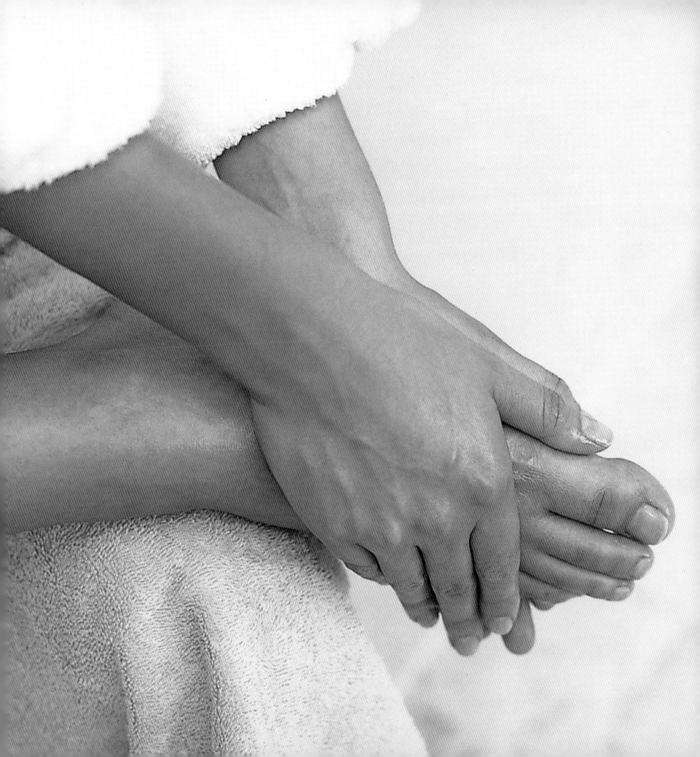

scented foot sprays

This spray and heat treatment is a sensual way to recharge the batteries. Its evocative aroma will revive flagging energy levels and lend your mood a quick boost.

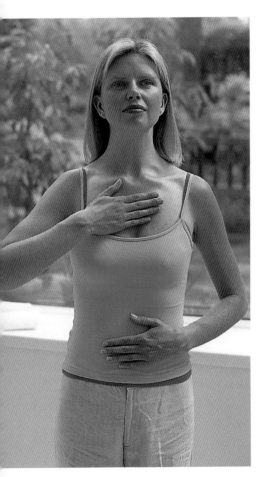

above *Foot sprays that harness natural flower perfumes can enliven the senses.*

The power of flowers to revive the spirits has been known throughout the centuries. Floral and herbal scents each have their own particular healing and restorative properties, but all have the ability to evoke an instant emotional reaction. Just walking past a flower shop or through a fragrant garden in springtime gives an instant boost.

jasmine euphoria spray

One of the most wonderful aromas in nature, jasmine has a euphoric effect and can lift your mood when you're feeling listless or depressed. You can use this jasmine oil spray at any time of year for an instant reminder of the beautiful things in life. The recipe makes about 30ml / 1fl oz, and can be sprayed on to the feet, used in conjunction with a warm compress, or both.

20ml / 4 tsp rose-water
5ml / 1 tsp orange flower water
5ml / 1 tsp vodka
7 drops jasmine essential oil
5 drops clary sage essential oil

1 Blend all the ingredients in a 30ml / 1fl oz spray bottle and shake. To use, place a large towel under your feet and spray your feet all over.

2 Now spray a small hand towel and wrap this around a hot-water bottle.
3 Place the hot-water bottle on the floor and rest your feet on it while you relax.

below *The scent of fresh jasmine flowers has a joyful effect on the senses, and is also said to have aphrodisiac qualities.*

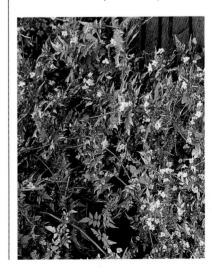

right *Apply this sleepy-time spray once in bed, so you can drift off straight away.*

sleepy-time oil spray

You can adapt the blend in this spray by changing the oils: a mixture of bergamot, clary sage, geranium and lemon, for example, will make a cleansing spray that is perfect for use after a workout.

25ml / 5 tsp grapeseed oil
25ml / 5 tsp almond oil
20ml / 4 tsp jojoba oil
10ml / 2 tsp rose-water
10ml / 2 tsp glycerine
20 drops each lavender and chamomile
   essential oils

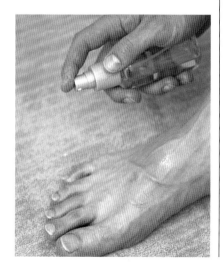

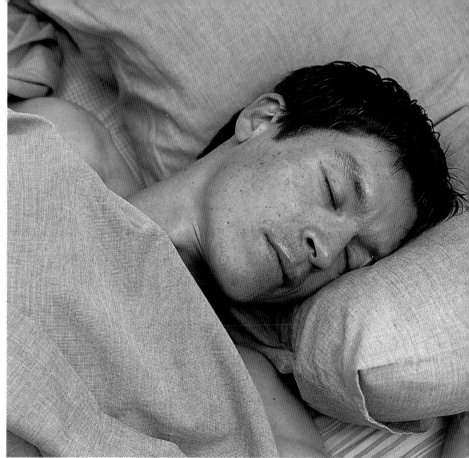

1 Mix the first five ingredients together, then stir in the essential oils, mixing together well.

2 Transfer to a clean 100ml / 3¹/₂fl oz spray bottle.

3 To apply, place a large towel beneath your feet and spray a large, clean tissue with the sleepy-time oil spray, then spray the top of your right foot.

4 Place the tissue on top of the foot, and use the sole of the left foot to wipe it across the surface of the right, gently massaging the oil into the skin.

5 Repeat this process on the left foot, so that the top and sole of both feet are lightly perfumed.

6 Now turn the right foot so that it is resting on its outer edge. Use the sole of the left foot to massage the sole of the right, then swap over.

7 To end, rub the soles of the feet on a towel to ensure they are free from any residue of oil. Lean back and close your eyes to relax, or if you are already in bed simply turn off the light, and get into a comfortable sleeping position.

index

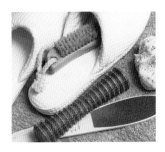

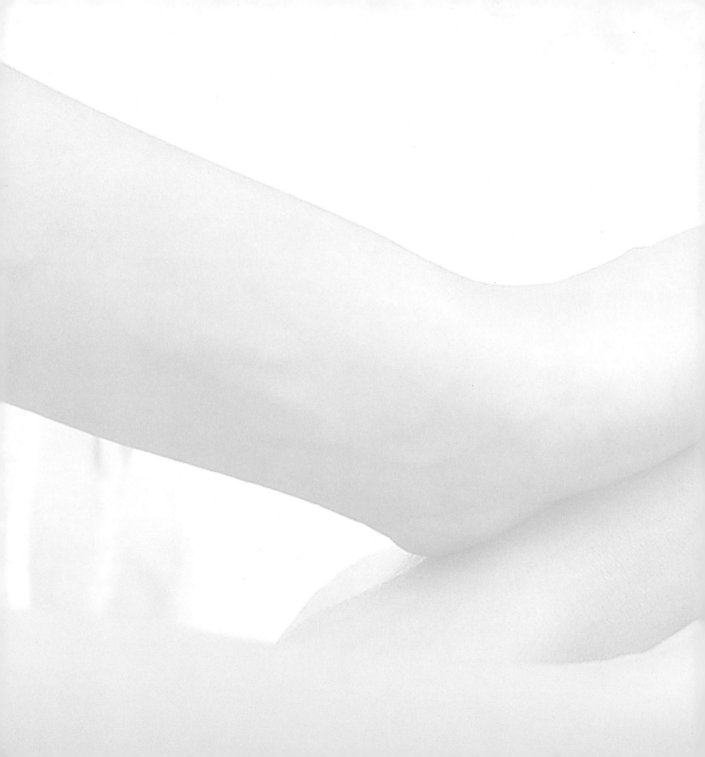